Domestic Production and Procurement of Medicines in Nigeria

Domestic Production and Procurement of Medicines in Nigeria:

Capabilities, Challenges and Prospects

By

Rachael Ayo-Lawal,
Caleb Adelowo,
Emmanuel Ejim-Eze,
Elizabeth Omimakinde,
Adesina Ayobami Oyewale,
Okechukwu Ukwuoma
and Wilson Erhun

Cambridge Scholars Publishing

Domestic Production and Procurement of Medicines in Nigeria:
Capabilities, Challenges and Prospects

By Rachael Ayo-Lawal, Caleb Adelowo, Emmanuel Ejim-Eze,
Elizabeth Omimakinde, Adesina Ayobami Oyewale,
Okechukwu Ukwuoma and Wilson Erhun

This book first published 2023

Cambridge Scholars Publishing

Lady Stephenson Library, Newcastle upon Tyne, NE6 2PA, UK

British Library Cataloguing in Publication Data
A catalogue record for this book is available from the British Library

ISBN (10): 1-5275-1271-1
ISBN (13): 978-1-5275-1271-9

National Centre for Technology Management (NACETEM)

An Agency of the Federal Ministry of Science, Technology & Innovation, Nigeria

Obafemi Awolowo University, Ile-Ife, Osun State, Nigeria.

About Nacetem

The National Centre for Technology Management (NACETEM) was established by the Federal Government of Nigeria in September 1992 as the Science and Technology (S&T) Policy Research and Training Centre under the National Planning Commission. Today, NACETEM operates as an agency of the Federal Ministry of Science, Technology and Innovation (FMSTI) and is vested with the mandate of training and developing middle- to high-level manpower, as well as engagement in policy research in the areas of Science, Technology and Innovation (STI) management for all tiers of government and the private sector. The Agency is located within the Obafemi Awolowo University, at the Ile-Ife campus. In the discharge of its mandates, the Agency provides knowledge support for the FMSTI and constitutes the software component of the Nation's STI system.

NACETEM's Vision Statement

To be an internationally recognized Centre of Excellence in Science, Technology and Innovation management for sustainable development

NACETEM's Mission Statement

To play a leading role in the build-up of expertise for effective management of Science, Technology and Innovation management and to actively engage in policy research, design, evaluation and review.

TABLE OF CONTENTS

LIST OF FIGURES

List of Tables

PREFACE

This document contains a summarised report of a survey of the Nigerian Pharmaceutical Industry titled "Towards a Competitive and Socially Inclusive Local Pharmaceutical Manufacturing in Nigeria". The study explored the following five thematic areas that are of relevance to the development of the industry in Nigeria:

1. Drug Affordability
2. Human Resources available for the Pharmaceutical Manufacturing Sector
3. Research and Development
4. Intellectual Property Rights and Technology Transfer & WHO Certification
5. Academia-Industry Linkages

The survey, which was conducted in 2019, was co-sponsored by the African Centre for Technology Studies (ACTS) Kenya, and the National Centre for Technology Management. The survey was supervised by Prof. W. Erhun of the Department of *Clinical Pharmacy and* Pharmacy Administration of the Obafemi Awolowo University, and Prof. Okechukwu Ukwuoma, the Director General/Chief Executive Officer (DG/CEO) of the National Centre for Technology Management (NACETEM), an Agency of Nigeria's Federal Ministry of Science, Technology & Innovation.

It is hoped that the implementation of policy interventions discussed in this book would enable the Nigerian Pharmaceutical Industry to develop along the path of excellence.

ACKNOWLEDGEMENTS

The National Centre for Technology Management (NACETEM) is grateful to the African Centre for Technology Studies (ACTS), Kenya, for awarding us the consultancy project titled "Building competitive and socially inclusive local pharmaceutical manufacturing in West Africa through enhancing research, innovation and intellectual property", on which this report is based.

The project team appreciates the support and cooperation of all individuals and organisations that have played key roles in the success of the survey. Most appreciated are key stakeholders whose responses formed the bedrock upon which this report stands. These include pharmaceutical firms, faculties of pharmacy, researchers in Nigerian universities and research institutes, and pharmaceutical associations and regulatory organisations. The interviewees include PCN, PSN, NAFDAC, NIPRD, NOTAP, BPP, PMG-MAN, AHAPN, RMRDC, the Food and Drugs Services Department of the Federal Ministry of Health, among others.

Finally, the project team is grateful to the DG/CEO of NACETEM, Engr (Prof.) Okechukwu Ukwuoma and the entire management for their support that enabled the project to be successful.

Thank you all.

Executive Summary

Healthcare for all can only be achieved when essential medicines are accessible and affordable to the general populace irrespective of their income status in a country or region. Access to affordable medicines remains a big challenge in developing countries, and Nigeria's case is worrisome because most people purchase their medicines out of pocket. Affordability poses a major barrier to accessing medicines for a reasonable percentage of the Nigerian population. Consequently, many Nigerians with chronic diseases do not access orthodox medications due to affordability issues; instead they use traditional medicines.

Previous studies in the early 2000s (FMoH-WHO, 2005) show that patients in Nigeria paid between 2 to 64 times the international reference prices for medicines at various health facilities in both the private and public sectors. These payments are mostly out-of-pocket expenditure (OOP); these make up about 95.9 per cent of all private expenditure on health in the country. The high cost of medicines in Nigeria is attributed to several factors including costly supply chains, poor government oversight, neglect/non-prioritization of the pharmaceutical industry, and loss of manufacturing capacity. The need to reposition pharmaceutical manufacturing in Nigeria necessitated this study.

This study investigated how issues such as the affordability/cost of medicines, human resources, research and development (R&D) activities, intellectual property protection, technology transfer, and government-academia-industry linkages affect pharmaceutical manufacturing and the entire pharmaceutical subsector in Nigeria. A mixed research method was adopted: this involved a desk review, key informant interviews and quantitative surveys of sampled pharmaceutical firms, research institutes and universities.

Our findings were not far from positions already established about the pharmaceutical industry in Nigeria. Serious challenges are confronting manufacturing in general; however, the high costs of importation of medicines and active pharmaceutical ingredients (API), and high OOP expenditures on healthcare constrain the social inclusion and competitiveness of drug manufacturing in Nigeria. The Nigerian pharmaceutical manufacturing sector is populated by small firms; and this impacts on their productivity, ability to conduct R&D, and overall technological capabilities. R&D involves high capital outlay and is a necessity for an industry such as pharmaceuticals. The size of these firms makes it impossible for them to mobilize the huge resources required for such R&D.

Moreover, the Nigerian health sector has been described by the United States Agency for International Development (USAID, 2021) as having one of the worst health indices in the world; and this could be partly attributed to the poor involvement of both the government and the private sector. Despite the opportunities, Nigerian pharmaceutical firms could neither capitalize on the Nigerian market nor benefit from the procurement system and the technologies developed from local R&D activities. The WHO earlier worked with eleven Nigerian pharmaceutical firms to achieve international good manufacturing practice (GMP) standards that would enable their products to become pre-qualified for WHO certification. Reports indicate that four of the companies have been pre-qualified by the WHO; however, one collapsed due largely to the huge capital involvement and the rigorous process of pursuing the qualification.

Results from our survey of Nigerian universities and schools of pharmacy reveal that about 40 per cent of the R&D undertaken by their researchers is mainly basic research, which may not be of immediate use to pharmaceutical firms. Lack of funds and non-availability of facilities/infrastructures including laboratories constrain their R&D efforts, including research and development of API. Self-sponsorships and government sponsorships are the major sources of funding for the R&D of the researchers. The study further reveals that high capital outlay, the WHO certification process, intellectual property issues, lack of incentives and the absence of a functional petrochemical industry also constrained the development of API in the country.

23 out of the 75 federal and state-owned universities offer pharmaceutical programs, and 21 of them are accredited by the Pharmaceutical Council of Nigeria (PCN) as of 2021. These 23 universities address the human resources needed in the Nigerian pharmaceutical industry. These institutions have produced well over 8,000 graduate pharmacists and about 800 postgraduates (Masters and Doctorate degree holders in Pharmaceutical Sciences) between 2014 and 2018.

The three research institutes that were covered in the study revealed that they have developed some products. The National Institute for Pharmaceutical Research and Development (NIPRD) developed Niprisan/Nicosan for the management of sickle cell anaemia and is in the process of developing other phytomedicines for the management of prevalent priority diseases; while the Nigeria Natural Medicine Development Agency (NNMDA) has developed various herbal therapies and nutritional supplements directed at health challenges such as diabetes, arthritis, topical dermatitis, erectile dysfunction and prostate enlargement, among others. The Nigerian Institute of Medical Research (NIMR) has been involved in testing for the efficacy of some drugs.

The successful development of Niprisan is an indicator of the potential and unexplored capabilities of the pharmaceutical industry in Nigeria. This calls for adequate funding for pharmaceutical R&D for the development of natural pharmaceutical resources, and challenges pharmaceutical firms to exploit local R&D outputs in their operations.

In conclusion, the Government of Nigeria has to give priority to the pharmaceutical industry for reasons of national security and the enhancement of local firms' performance.

LIST OF ACRONYMS

ACPN	Association of Community Pharmacists of Nigeria
ACTS	African Centre for Technology Studies
AHAPN	Association of Hospital and Administrative Pharmacists of Nigeria
API	Active Pharmaceutical Ingredient
ARVs	Antiretrovirals
BPP	Bureau for Public Procurement
FMoH	Federal Ministry of Health
FMST	Federal Ministry of Science and Technology
GMP	Good Manufacturing Practices
HIV/AIDS	Human Immunodeficiency Virus/Acquired Immunodeficiency Syndrome
IP	Intellectual Property
IPR	Intellectual Property Rights
IPTTO	Intellectual Property Technology Transfer Office
NAFDAC	National Agency for Food and Drug Administration and Control
NOTAP	National Office for Technology Acquisition and Protection
NAIP	Nigerian Association of Industrial Pharmacists
NHIS	National Health Insurance Scheme
NIMR	Nigeria Institute of Medical Research
NIPRD	National Institute for Pharmaceutical Research and Development
NNMDA	Nigeria Natural Medicine Development Agency
NUC	National Universities Commission
PCN	Pharmacists Council of Nigeria
PMG-MAN	Pharmaceutical Manufacturing Group of Manufacturers Association of Nigeria
PSN	Pharmaceutical Society of Nigeria
RMRDC	Raw Materials Research and Development Council
R&D	Research and Development
SHESTCO	SHEDA Science and Technology Complex
SON	Standards Organisation of Nigeria
TETFUND	Tertiary Education Trust Fund

TRIPS	Trade-Related Aspects Intellectual Property
UHC	Universal Health Coverage
UNESCO	United Nations Educational, Scientific and Cultural Organization
UNIDO	United Nations Industrial Development Organization
WAPCP	West African Postgraduate College of Pharmacists
WHO	World Health Organization
WIPO	World Intellectual Property Organization

CHAPTER ONE

INTRODUCTION

Health is one of the major human development indices and the need for Universal Health Coverage (UHC) was acknowledged in Sustainable Development Goal (SDG) 3, which aims to *"Ensure healthy lives and promote well-being for all at all ages"*[1]. To achieve this goal, it is important to provide quality health care to the populace through the establishment of healthcare infrastructure, the recruitment of qualified personnel and the provision of adequate, affordable, and quality medicines. However, the provision of adequate, affordable, and quality health care to the population remains a major challenge for governments in many African countries including Nigeria, a country with a high burden of tropical diseases, and consequently, with poor health indicator indices. For instance, the Health Access Quality (HAQ) Index (GDB, 2016) ranked Nigeria 187 out of 195 countries in 2018,[2] while the Global Health Security Index was estimated to be only 32.3, ranking Nigeria 130 out of 195 countries in the year 2019.[3]

Inadequate access to essential drugs and other healthcare commodities has been identified as having negative impacts on people's health in most developing countries (UNIDO, 2011). To address this challenge in Nigeria, the Nigerian Government has been targeting the availability of effective, affordable, safe and good quality medicines at all times and in all sectors of the health care system. To achieve this goal, a policy thrust of the government that is contained in the National Drug Policy is to ensure adequate supplies of drugs (FMoH, 2018). The first National Drug Policy that was published in 1990 and the revised version of 2005 targeted the availability of drugs as stated above. However, decades after the first Policy was launched, many of the set targets are yet to be realized.

---

[1] https://www.un.org/sustainabledevelopment/health/

[2] https://businessday.ng/health/article/nigerias-health-care-system-ranks-187th-globally/

[3] https://www.ghsindex.org/wp-content/uploads/2019/10/2019-Global-Health-Security-Index.pdf

As noted earlier, the Nigerian health sector has been described as having one of the poorest health indices in the world and this has been partly attributed to underfunding of the sector by the government. For instance, between 2009 and 2018, the cumulative budget of the Federal Government of Nigeria (FGN) for 10 years was N55.19 trillion. Of this amount, the health sector was allocated N2.51 trillion, which is 4.55 per cent. This percentage is far below the 13 per cent that was recommended by the World Health Organisation (WHO) and the 15 per cent that the African Union recommended[4] (Obasanjo, 2018). The low budgetary allocation to the health sector notwithstanding, most of the budget is spent on personnel costs. Consequently, the health of most Nigerians remains poor and the country remains fraught with poverty, diseases and malnutrition.

Access to medicines is an integral component of Universal Health Coverage (UHC). Target 3.8 of the Sustainable Development Goals (SDGs) specifically declares *"Access to safe, effective, quality and affordable essential medicines and vaccines for all"* (UN, 2015). This declaration and target underscore the importance of a robust and reliable pharmaceutical sector in any economy, given its prominent role in the health status and general well-being of the citizens. In Nigeria, there is a continuous growing demand for safe, effective and affordable medicines, but weak local pharmaceutical manufacturing capacity is making the country depend largely on imported medicines.

According to UNIDO (2011), the installed capacity utilization of about 120 local drug manufacturers that existed in Nigeria as at the time of compiling the report was about 40 per cent. This level of production was only able to satisfy 25 per cent of the local demand for drugs, while imports, mainly from Asian countries (especially India and China) accounted for the remaining 75 per cent. As of 2013, pharmaceutical imports in Nigeria amounted to about US $481 million (Gumel, 2014) and increased to about US $1.45 billion in 2019.[5]

Pharmaceutical industrial firms in Nigeria are confronted with several constraints that make local products more expensive when compared with imported ones. The firms operate with high production costs as a result of the high cost of inputs, poor infrastructure, inconsistent local and regional

---

[4] Obasanjo, O. (2018) Vanguard, 8th July. https://www.vanguardngr.com/2018/07/nigeria-has-some-of-the-worst-health-indices-in-the-world-obasanjo/

[5] https://tradingeconomics.com/nigeria/imports/pharmaceutical-products

tariffs, difficult access to foreign exchange as well as the devaluation of the Naira (NGN), the Nigerian currency, in the international market, thereby rendering the cost of imported raw materials high.

Another threat confronting Nigeria's Pharmaceutical Sector is drug price control. UNIDO (2011) reveals that prices of health products in the market are high and most Nigerians cannot afford them. Therefore, given the high prices of drugs, rising health care spending, and a larger percentage of the Nigerian population purchasing drugs through out-of-pocket expenses, the goal of making drugs accessible and affordable remains unrealised.

The aforementioned challenges result in low-capacity utilization, and a reduction in domestic drug production in Nigeria. Beyond policy reversals and inconsistency, there are also the problems of low patronage of drugs made in Nigeria. This is worsened by problems of unregulated drug distribution channels that have promoted illicit markets in tandem with fake and substandard products. UNIDO (2011) noted that manufacturers' products are routinely faked and sold at lower prices than genuine products; consequently, local drug manufacturers are losing a significant share of the drug market in Nigeria to illicit drug dealers. The poor performance of the pharmaceutical industry has manifested itself in the poor health indicators of the country. With the high population of Nigeria, which makes the country a big market for pharmaceutical products, reliance on the importation of bulk drugs and active pharmaceutical ingredients (API) would not be sufficiently beneficial to the national economy, and it is not a reliable option for the supply of medicines to citizens of the country, as the constancy and adequacy of their supply cannot be guaranteed. This may render Nigerian citizens vulnerable to interruption of the supply of medicines. To prevent this from occurring, there is a need to promote domestic drug manufacturing.

Many authors have written about the Nigerian Pharmaceutical Industry. For instance, UNIDO (2011) published a profile of the industry as of 2011. The publication, which was the report of a project on strengthening the local production of essential generic drugs in the country, provided a comprehensive picture of the status and operating environment of the pharmaceutical sector in Nigeria. The publication was also designed to assist stakeholders with the necessary information for discussions on how local production fits into the strategy for an improved supply of medicines.

To enable us to assess the Nigerian Pharmaceutical Sectoral Ecosystem with a view to build an inclusive, formidable and competitive local pharmaceutical manufacturing industry, this study gathered information on diverse aspects of the industry including: the status of Research and Development (R&D), available human resources, capabilities for the production of Active Pharmaceutical Ingredients (API), and issues associated with intellectual property and technology transfer in the sector. The study also obtained information on various challenges confronting the industry. The role and extent of interaction between the pharmaceutical firms, university pharmacy faculties, the Nigerian government and its agencies, and other stakeholders in the Nigerian Pharmaceutical Sector Ecosystem were also obtained.

Research Context: Pharmaceutical Industry in Nigeria

Nigeria has the biggest and one of the most rapidly growing pharmaceutical industries and also the largest market for pharmaceutical products in Africa. The country has over 200 registered pharmaceutical firms, of which about 120 are involved in the manufacturing of medicinal products (UNIDO, 2011). Among these firms, nine are listed on the Nigerian Stock Exchange; and five of these listed companies are indigenous. The nine quoted firms are responsible for about 58 per cent of the manufactured pharmaceutical products in Nigeria (AUC/UNDO, 2012; Gumel, 2014; Ugbam and Okoro, 2017). While most pharma firms operating in Nigeria are affiliated with multinational companies, others are either privately or publicly owned.

The Nigerian pharmaceutical industry is a major player among the countries of the Economic Community of West African States (ECOWAS), and it has the potential to be a leader in the production and distribution of pharmaceuticals to Sub-Saharan Africa. Nine of the pharmaceutical firms operating in Nigeria currently export their products to various ECOWAS countries (Obukohwo et al., 2018). Furthermore, UNIDO (2011) reports that health products produced in Nigeria account for about 60 per cent of all drug consumption in the ECOWAS countries.

The estimated value of the Nigerian pharmaceutical industry in 2016 was US $9.4bn and was projected to rise to $13.2bn by 2020, while the market was estimated to be worth about $3.0bn (UNECA, 2020). This high potential demand notwithstanding, the Nigerian pharmaceutical industry is not able to fully satisfy the Nigerian market; consequently, the country has to depend on importation. Probably, the poor performance of the industry is one of the factors responsible for the poor health indices of Nigerian citizens. Ugbam and Okoro (2017) noted that Nigeria does not feature among the 17 notable pharma growth markets in the sector. Worse still, imports of pharmaceutical products to Nigeria rose from US $481m in 2013

(Gumel, 2014) to $1.45 billion in 2021[6]. This poor performance of the local pharmaceutical industry in providing the drugs needed for the Nigerian market, and the consequential importation to cover the deficit, points to the need for stakeholders in the industry to promote local pharmaceutical manufacturing companies to improve on their capacity utilization.

Scope of the Study

The main issues covered in this survey were affordability of medicines, human resource development and its availability for the pharmaceutical manufacturing sector, research and development (R&D) activities in support of industrial production, intellectual property rights and technology transfer activities on pharmaceutical products. Others are WHO certification for medicines that are produced in Nigeria for export and research-industry interaction within the Nigeria Pharmaceutical System. The study specifically obtained information on the factors influencing the productivity of Nigeria's pharmaceutical manufacturers and the roles of key stakeholders within the system. The information was collected with the aim of designing appropriate policy interventions that could help build a robust local pharmaceutical manufacturing industry in Nigeria.

Methodology

The research design adopted for the study included a desk review for relevant information, surveys covering pharmaceutical firms, research institutes and universities with schools of pharmacy and pharmacy-related programmes, and key informant interviews.

A. Desk Review

The desk-based component of the study involved a review of relevant academic literature on the current position of the pharmaceutical industry in Nigeria. These included journals, books, reports, working papers, and the grey literature. In addition, several secondary sources of data including global bodies (WHO, UNIDO, etc.) and the publications of relevant national government ministries, departments and agencies (MDAs) were accessed for information.

---

[6] https://tradingeconomics.com/nigeria/imports/pharmaceutical-products

B. Quantitative Surveys

Three set of structured questionnaires were designed and used to obtain information from three groups of respondents: research institutes, university pharmaceutical researchers, and pharmaceutical firms. The questionnaires included both close-ended and open-ended questions.

Sample and Sampling Techniques

- The research institutes covered were: the Nigeria Natural Medicine Development Agency (NNMDA), National Institute for Pharmaceutical Research and Development (NIPRD) and Nigerian Institute of Medical Research (NIMR).
- 55 pharmaceutical manufacturing firms, spread across seven states in five geographical zones of the country were selected for the study. The firms included major players in the industry that were purposefully selected, while the rest were randomly selected. Figure 1.1 shows states with manufacturing pharma firms that were covered. One copy of the questionnaire was completed by each firm.
- All the 21 universities with faculties of pharmacy were covered in the survey. One set of the questionnaires was administered on the dean of the Faculty and the Heads of the following departments in the faculties: Department of Pharmacognosy, Pharmacology, Pharmaceutics, and Pharmaceutical Chemistry and other similar departments.

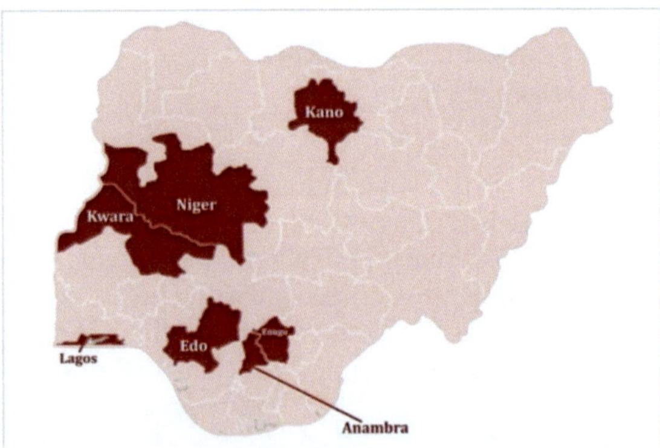

Figure 1.1: Map of Nigeria Showing States Spread of Manufacturing Pharma Firms Captured in the Study

C. Key Informant Interviews

The study collected data from relevant stakeholders with interviews conducted with key informants within the Nigerian Pharmaceutical Industry to address the identified research questions on the roles each of them is playing in the Industry. The interviews were conducted with the Director-General/Chief Executive Officers (D-G/CEO) of the organisations or their nominees, using interview guides focussing on the activities of the organisation in question. The interview guides sought to obtain information on the role of each organisation in strengthening and enhancing the performance of the Nigerian pharma sector, as well as their interaction with other players in the industry. The majority of the interviews were conducted face-to-face, while some were conducted over the telephone. The Nigeria Government organizations covered were: the Department of Food and Drug Services of the Federal Ministry of Health, Raw Materials Research and Development Council (RMRDC), National Agency for Food and Drug Administration and Control (NAFDAC), National Institute for Pharmaceutical Research and Development (NIPRD), Nigeria Natural Medicine Development Agency (NNMDA) and Nigerian Institute of Medical Research (NIMR).

The non-governmental organizations that were covered included: the Pharmaceutical Manufacturing Group of the Manufacturers Association of Nigeria (PMG-MAN), Pharmacists Council of Nigeria (PCN), Pharmaceutical Society of Nigeria (PSN), Association of Hospital and Administrative Pharmacists of Nigeria (AHAPN), Association of Community Pharmacists of Nigeria (ACPN), Nigerian Association of Industrial Pharmacists (NAIP), Nigerian Representatives of Overseas Pharmaceutical Manufacturers (NIROPHARM) and the West African Postgraduate College of Pharmacists (WAPCP). All interviews were audio recorded, and they were later transcribed by trained personnel. The responses were thereafter used as appropriate in the compilation of the results. Efforts to conduct face-to-face or telephone interviews with officials of three of the organisations were futile, consequently, information that was relevant to the study regarding the activities of these organizations, which was obtained from other reliable sources, was used in the report.

Data Collection and Analyses

The three sets of questionnaires that were administered to the research institutes were successfully retrieved from them, while 69 out of the 105 copies of questionnaire that were administered to the universities were retrieved, representing a 66 per cent retrieval rate. Out of the 55 copies of questionnaire that were administered to the industrial firms, 32 were retrieved giving a response rate of about 59 per cent for the firms. The list of firms that returned completed questionnaires is presented in Appendix 2, and the number of questionnaires retrieved from each geographical zone is as follows:

- South East: 11
- South South: 3
- South West: 14
- North West: 2
- North Central: 2

Data collected were analyzed using descriptive analysis with the aid of the Statistical Package for Social Sciences (SPSS) tool.

Study Challenges

The researchers experienced some constraints in the course of data collection, especially data collection from firms. Efforts to gain access to the premises of many pharma firms proved abortive: some even claimed non-acceptance of questionnaires as company policy; while some firms that collected the questionnaires did not return them. A similar situation was experienced among the academia, as some of them did not return their questionnaires. Another challenge that was encountered was that some firms claimed they are no longer involved in drug production and so were excluded from the list, while others had either relocated or folded up.

Results and Discussion

The next five chapters of this report are used to present the results from the surveys and key informant interviews to provide a holistic view of the Nigerian Pharmaceutical Sector under the following five main themes:

1. Affordability;
2. Research and Development;
3. Intellectual Property Rights Issues, Technology Transfer and WHO Certification;
4. Interaction Within Nigeria's Pharmaceutical Industry;
5. Human Resource Development for the Pharmaceutical manufacturing sector.

CHAPTER TWO

AFFORDABILITY OF DRUGS IN NIGERIA: ISSUES AND CHALLENGES

EMMANUEL E. EJIM-EZE

Introduction

Healthcare for all can only be achieved when essential medicines are accessible and affordable to the general populace irrespective of their income status in a country or region. Access to medicine is described as "the percentage of population that has access to a minimum list of 20 essential medicines, which are continuously available and affordable at a health facility or medicines outlet, within one hour's walk from the patient's home".[1] WHO (2018) reported that access to medicines is a multidimensional problem in view of the rising prices of new medicines and persisting problems of medicine shortages, among other reasons. The World Medicines Situation (WHO, 2004) and Jitta *et al*. (2003) estimated that about half of the population in Africa lack regular access to essential medicines. Consequently, having access to quality affordable medicines remains a big challenge in many developing countries, Nigeria included (DFID, 2004; Nyanwura and Esena, 2013; Ekeigwe, 2019).

Previous studies of medicine prices in Nigeria indicated that 90 per cent of Nigerians (who live below the income level of US $2 per day, as well as government workers who earn a minimum wage of US $1.4 per day) cannot afford medicines (McIntyre *et al.,* 2006; Wambebe and Ochekpe, 2011). Affordability poses a major barrier to access to medicines for a reasonable population of Nigerians, and some segments of the population with chronic diseases do not take medications due to affordability issues (FMST, 2011). This barrier is based on the fact that out-of-pocket expenditure (OOP) makes up about 95.9 per cent of all private expenditure on health in Nigeria.

[1] https://rho.emro.who.int/Metadata/availability-of-selected-essential-medicines

The prevalence of OOP in Nigeria has continued to rise since the year 2000, and was 77.22 per cent of the health expenditure in 2017 (World Bank, 2020). This 2017 value for Nigeria's OOP was double the sub-Saharan African average of 35.54 per cent for the year.

Prices of Medicines in Nigeria

Drug prices in Nigeria are set mostly by market forces, with government tariffs, taxes and distribution mark-ups accounting for a significant proportion of the final price. Prices vary between outlets, facilities and types of products, with generic drugs priced much higher than their equivalents in neighbouring countries. A national survey on medicine prices was undertaken in 2004 by the Federal Ministry of Health (FMoH) in collaboration with the World Health Organization (WHO), the UK's Department for International Development (DFID), the European Union and Health Action International (FMoH-WHO, 2002, FMoH, 2010). The results of the survey revealed the following:

1. Patients pay between 2-64 times the international reference prices for medicines at various health facilities in both the private and public sectors;
2. Prices in the public sector were almost identical to those in the private pharmacies;
3. Private health clinics charge about 184 per cent more than public health facilities and about 193 per cent more than private retail pharmacies;
4. Innovator brands cost between 2-7 times the lowest priced generic equivalents;
5. Affordability was largely dependent on the choice of therapeutic class, product or sector from which the medicine was purchased. For example: - "A worker would pay 0.7 days' wages to treat an infection with amoxicillin and pay an additional 18.8 days' wages when using ceftriaxone injection to treat the same infection";
6. While innovator branded medicines compared well with prices in other countries, generic medicines were up to 825 per cent more expensive in Nigeria when compared to seven other countries;
7. Medicine prices are made up of such components as government tariffs and taxes, as well as mark-ups for distribution, which account for a significant proportion of what patients pay for medicines. Mark–ups by the importers, distributors and retailers were found to be up to 900 per cent the manufacturers' price.

The high cost of medicines in Nigeria is due to a costly supply chain and poor government oversight. This cost has hindered a large proportion of Nigeria's population from being able to afford medicines, even when the medicines are available. The issue of the non-affordability of medicines is addressed in the revised National Drug Policy that authorises the Bureau for Public Procurement to facilitate bulk purchase of medicine for government hospitals, and the National Health Insurance Scheme that offers healthcare subsidies to its enrollees.

Drug Procurement in Nigeria

The Federal and State Governments in Nigeria are making efforts to make drugs affordable to the populace through the procurement schemes they have initiated. According to the official that represented the Federal Ministry of Health for the key informant interview, the current practice in Nigeria with respect to procurement of medicine by the Federal Government is the Drug Revolving Fund, which is a key component of the Essential Medicine Program of the Government. The officer disclosed that:

> A key component of the Essential Medicine Program of the Government is the Drug Revolving Fund (DRF) Scheme, through which a dedicated pool of fund for the purpose of procuring essential medicines is recycled. This policy of the Government ensures that essential medicines are affordable, accessible, efficacious and safe. The drugs are purchased directly from the manufacturers or importers so that the long chain of movement is side-lined, because at each junction of the chain there is inbuilt profit margin. The principle behind this direct procurement of essential medicine is that the Government invest once and the operators of the scheme manage the fund, which they recycle without going back to the Government. The drugs are sold with a little margin so that they would be affordable to the generality of the populace.

The Public Procurement Act of 2007 (FGN 2007) the Nigeria's National Drug Policy (FMoH-WHO, 2005), and the Executive Order 003 (FGN, 2017) are policy instruments through which the FGN emphasized the need to patronize made-in-Nigeria goods. Beside the issue of making essential medicine affordable, the Public Procurement Act of 2007 regulates the procurement of drugs by Government agencies in Nigeria. Below is a description of the activities of the Bureau of Public Procurement.

Public Procurement Act 2007

The procurement process is a major determinant of the availability and affordability of controlled medicines in government hospitals. To encourage patronage of locally produced goods the Federal Government of Nigeria passed the Public Procurement Act 2007 (FGN, 2007) which established the Bureau of Public Procurement (BPP). The Act empowers the BPP to oversee all procurement processes in all public and government agencies in Nigeria. These include the procurement of goods (including medicines), services and works. The objectives of the Bureau are harmonized with existing government policies and practices on public procurement and aim to ensure probity, accountability and transparency in the procurement process; the establishment of pricing standards and benchmarks; and the attainment of transparency, competitiveness, cost effectiveness and professionalism in the public sector procurement system. The BPP also has the power to review all procurement transactions to ensure compliance with the provisions of the Public Procurement Act and to debar any supplier, contractor or service provider who contravenes any provision of the Act.

The 2007 Act stipulates Nigerian Government Policy in support of preference for supplies of domestic products and services for Government projects. The Act empowers the BPP to grant a margin of preference in the evaluation of tenders when comparing bids from domestic companies with those from foreign firms or when comparing tenders from domestic suppliers offering goods manufactured locally with those offering goods manufactured abroad. Where a procuring entity intends to allow domestic preferences, the bidding documents must clearly indicate that preference will be given to domestic suppliers and contractors and must also provide the information required to establish the eligibility of a bid for such preference. Margins of preference shall apply only to tenders under international competitive bidding. The Act further empowers the BPP to set the limits, compute the margins of preference and determine the contents of goods manufactured locally, from time the time.

Government Procurement Policy (in BPP) stipulates that 70 per cent of essential medicines that are procured by the Government should be procured locally. However, it is not certain if the people implementing the policies are following its dictates. A comment from one of the key informants suggested that efforts are being intensified on advocacy to remind government agencies and MDAs to abide by the policies and patronize medicines that are manufactured in Nigeria. There is also the need to review the NHIS Policy to lay more emphases on the use of locally manufactured medicines.

National Health Insurance Scheme

The National Health Insurance Scheme was officially launched in June 2005 (Adewole et al., 2015)), with a presidential directive that there should be universal coverage by 2015. The aim of the scheme is to provide affordable healthcare services to Nigerians. The scheme starts with the formal sector comprising the Public Sector, the Organized Private Sector and the Armed Forces, Police and other Uniformed Services; thereafter, the scheme is expected to be extended to the informal sector. The scheme obliges all employees of the formal sector to contribute 15 per cent of their salary (5 per cent is provided by employees and the remainder by employers) to Health Maintenance Organizations (HMOs), which will arrange for the necessary healthcare for the participants. Contributions are earnings-related. For the Public (federal) sector participants, the employer pays 3.25 per cent while the employee pays 1.75 per cent, representing 5 per cent of the employee's consolidated salary. For the private sector participants and those in other tiers of Government, the employer pays 10 per cent while the employee pays 5 per cent, representing 15 per cent of the employee's basic salary. However, the employer may decide to pay the entire contribution. The contributions paid cover healthcare benefits for the employee, one spouse and four biological children below the age of 18 years. More dependents or children above the age of 18 could also be covered on the payment of additional contributions by the principal beneficiary as determined by NHIS.

The NHIS scheme, in compliance with a presidential directive was expected to have achieved universal coverage by 2015. However, this is still far from being achieved. Since its inception, the majority of Nigerians are yet to be enrolled into the scheme, except for Federal public servants and their families, who make up a large percentage of subscribers to the scheme. Therefore, the coverage of NHIS is restricted to a relatively small number of people out of Nigeria's large population profile. Furthermore, the scheme is yet to be extended to people engaged in the small- and medium-sized enterprises and the entire informal sector in Nigeria that constitutes the larger percentage of the population.

State and cooperative organizations health insurance schemes are also being established in different locations in Nigeria to bridge the coverage gaps left by the NHIS. As of 2019, 19 states are at various stages of the implementation of their health insurance schemes (PWC, 2019). Like the NHIS, a government agency is established for the implementation and management of each of the state-operated schemes. The State Governments commit funds to the scheme to offer premiums for the poor and vulnerable in their various states (a map of Nigeria showing states that have Health Insurance Schemes is presented in Figure 2.1). However, there are doubts about further implementation and development of the State Health Insurance Scheme (SHIS) because the Nigeria Medical Association (NMA) believed that the capitation paid by NHIS (N750) in Nigeria for patients is poor, yet some states were trying to offer less than N500 to treat their citizens (Onyeji, 2018). NHIS has encountered multiple challenges during the 13 years since its implementation and the NMA felt that issues should not be compounded by the introduction of SHIS. As a result, NMA has since asked its members to distance from SHIS; while the issue of poor disbursements of funds is still burning.

The public sector contribution to healthcare has been rising since the introduction of the NHIS. The intervention of PBPP has facilitated bulk purchase of medicines and other products needed for the scheme; thereby lowering the cost of medicines in the market, while at the same time boosting the scheme. The Federal Government procures drugs for the Federal University Teaching Hospitals and the Federal Medical Centres that are at the tertiary levels; while state and local governments cater for the healthcare at state hospitals and primary healthcare centres respectively. This fragmentation of drug procurement also affects the affordability, quality and quantity of drugs dispensed at each level of healthcare in Nigeria.

Besides government procurement, Nigeria has been benefiting from donor medicine procurement. A major foreign source of funds for procurement of medicines in Nigeria is The Global Fund. The Fund provided Nigeria with various amounts to fight malaria, HIV/AIDS and Tuberculosis (TB) between 2005 and 2009. In 2006, the Fund threatened to suspend the funding of projects in Nigeria because the country failed to meet targets on drug access and "transparency", but later, allocated some funds to Nigeria in the 2017-2019 Allocation Periods; and disbursed US $76.6m for HIV/AIDS, $1.48m for TB/HIV; and $2.11m for Resilient and Sustainable Systems for Health (RSSH) (The Global Fund 2019). Presently, the Nigerian government mostly procures first line ARV drugs while development partners take care of second- and third-line drugs.

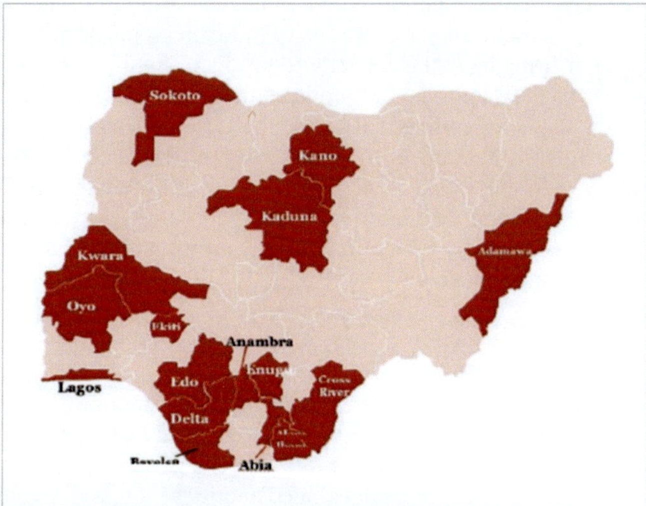

Figure 2.1: Map of Nigeria Showing States Having Health Insurance Schemes
Source: (PwC, 2019)

Over the years, the Nigerian government has targeted provision of adequate supplies of drugs that are effective, affordable, safe and of good quality at all times and in all sectors of the health care system. These are contained in Nigeria's first National Drug Policy document published in 1990, revised in 2005, and currently under revision from 2018 (FMoH, 2018). Decades after the first document was produced, many of the set targets are yet to be realized, the budgetary expenditures in the health sector notwithstanding. The health of most Nigerians remains poor. The country remains fraught with poverty, diseases and malnutrition.

National Drug Policy

The problem of the price of medicine is addressed in the revised National Drug Policy of 2005, which set out to present acceptable determinants of medicine prices in all sectors, thereby making medicines more affordable. Furthermore, one of the activities of the Bureau for Public Procurement has been facilitating bulk purchases of medicines and other products, consequently reducing the cost of medicines in the market. One factor that could lead to further reduction in the price of medicines in Nigeria is the increment in capacity utilization of the local manufacturers of the products, which was reported to be only 40% by UNIDO (2011). Nigerian pharmaceutical firms may not be able to revamp their idle capacities on their own; hence, government support could be needed. Therefore, government policies aiming to reduce the importation of those medicines which Nigerian pharmaceutical firms have the capacity to produce should be designed and implemented. In the same manner, policies that would enable the firms to increase their capacity utilization should be designed and implemented. Although Presidential Executive Order 003 reads "*All Ministries, Departments and Agencies (MDAs) of the Federal Government of Nigeria shall grant preference to local manufacturers of goods and service providers in their procurement of goods and services*", an informant doubted its full implementation in practice.

National Health Policy

The Federal Ministry of Health is responsible for implementing the National Health Policy (NHP). Nigeria has implemented three NHPs, the first from 1988, the second from 2004, and the third, which is the latest, from 2016. The 1988 and 2004 polices were developed at critical stages of evolution of the Health Sector system in Nigeria and had a significant impact on the national health landscape.

The 2004 NHP attempted to address the inadequacies of the Nigerian Health Sector by identifying seven priority areas and recommending improvements in the following areas:

i. Increased funding of the health system;
ii. Expansion of information communication technologies in the Department of Food and Drug Services of the Federal Ministry of Health;
iii. Promotion of local production of essential medicines;
iv. Improved consumer awareness;
v. Promotion of effective partnership, collaboration and coordination;
vi. Revitalisation of the primary health care (PHC) system; and
vii. Strengthening of regulatory mechanisms.

The 2016 policy was drafted to key into the Sustainable Development Goals (SDGs). The 2016 Policy has a framework and strategies that could enable Nigeria to achieve universal health coverage. The objective of the new policy is to provide support and strengthen the national health system in addition to providing financial risks protection to all Nigerians, especially the poor and most vulnerable groups.

In specific terms, the NHP of 2016 intended to achieve the following goals:

- Revise, update and implement the National Drug Policy, the National Essential Medicine list, the Nigerian Supply Chain policy for pharmaceuticals and other healthcare products, and the National Quality Assurance Policy for Medicines and other health products;
- Promote the local production of high-quality medicines, vaccines, therapeutic foods, commodities and other health technologies;
- Facilitate public/private partnerships in the production of medicines and vaccines;
- Support more local drug manufacturers to attain the WHO-prequalification status;
- Strengthen existing systems for effective monitoring, surveillance and evaluation in the logistics channel for health care delivery; and
- Strengthen relevant regulatory bodies (NAFDAC and SON) to reduce the supply of fake and substandard medicines, vaccines, commodities and other technologies for health care delivery.

Impact of Subsidy on the Development of Local Pharmaceutical Industry

According to UNIDO (2011), healthcare subsidy policies are expected to affect the growth of the local pharmaceutical industry in Nigeria. The Public Procurement Act 2007 gave preference to domestic suppliers and those offering goods manufactured locally, compared with those offering foreign manufactured goods. Drug manufacturers in Nigeria are up against several constraints, including low capacity utilization, under capitalization, weak financial base, high production costs as a result of the high cost of inputs, poor infrastructure, difficulty in meeting WHO prequalification criteria, low level or obsolete technologies, high interest rates and unstable demand. The fluctuations in demand are a reflection of the prevailing low purchasing power of the population and the fact that government purchases of medicines are irregular and payments are sometimes delayed.

The issue of the affordability of medicines is somehow tied to local production of pharmaceuticals in Nigeria. The Nigerian pharmaceutical manufacturing sector is populated by small firms, and only nine out of over 130 registered pharmaceutical companies were listed on the Nigerian stock exchange as of 2014 (Gumel, 2014). Consequently, the small size of the firms impacts on their productivity, research and development (R&D), as well as on their overall technological capabilities. According to the World Bank Business Monitor International (Ugbam and Okoro, 2007), the combined total output of the Nigerian pharmaceutical industry is US $1.28 billion, and this is approximately the output of a medium-sized firm elsewhere in the world.

Records show that patent registries of Nigeria and other West African countries grant high percentages of the patents they register to foreign applicants. The 1999-2002 data shows that out of the 2,544 patents issued, 1,458 were granted to foreign and 986 to local applicants; and it was reported that some of the patents are being exploited by Nigerian pharmaceutical manufacturing firms under license from foreign owners (Adewopo, 2011). Obviously, not much R&D is conducted among Nigerian pharmaceutical manufacturing firms, and this is mostly linked to their small size, which makes it practically impossible for them to mobilize the huge resources required for R&D. Therefore, the companies mostly produce products under licenses from foreign pharmaceutical firms. This arrangement affects the prices of pharmaceuticals produced in Nigeria, and consequently their affordability.

Previously, the Nigerian government along with other members of the ECOWAS adopted a Common External Tariff (CET). The CET had a four-band structure which included: 0 per cent (for products with social significance, such as medicines), 5 per cent (for necessities and raw materials), 10 per cent (for intermediate goods) and 20 per cent (for finished consumer goods). However, the CET was later reviewed when it was realised to be unfavourable to the local pharmaceutical industry, because some production also takes place in other ECOWAS countries. Presently, the importation of raw materials attracts 0 per cent VAT, while VAT on importation of finished products is between 10 and 20 per cent VAT to discourage it.

Beyond procurement, tariff and other financial incentives, the Nigerian government also provides necessary support to facilitate the production of pharmaceutical API in Nigeria, though presently pharmaceutical firms import API to produce drugs in the country. Production of API is a capital-intensive endeavour that requires many resources – huge capital, good infrastructure, political commitment, and a well-designed programme to achieve it. Making Nigeria's petrochemical industry functional would be a good beginning, as many of the products from that sector are needed in the synthesis of several drugs. To encourage local production of API, a key informant recommended that the FGN should establish an API Park possibly within any of the Free Trade Zones, where companies that intend to produce API can establish their manufacturing plants. In the words of the informant, “such Park models have been used by countries such as Bangladesh, India and Ethiopia to develop their API industries”.

The window of opportunity available through TRIPS flexibilities allowed the least developed countries to locally produce generic medicines until 2016 (Berger *et al.,* 2010); however, countries with poor technological capability could not utilize the opportunity. A generic drug is a medication that is created to be the same as an already marketed brand-name drug in dosage form, safety, strength, route of administration, quality, performance characteristics, and intended use. These similarities help to demonstrate bioequivalence, which means that *a generic medicine works in the same way and provides the same clinical benefit as the brand-name medicine.* In other words, a generic medicine is an equal substitute for its brand-name counterpart (USFDA, 2021). Generic drugs by firms that differ from the branded drugs producers are usually produced at a much lower cost, thereby making their prices lower and more affordable than the original brand-name product.

Nigeria failed to utilise the opportunity of TRIPS flexibilities to enter the league of generic medicine producers. According to a key informant interviewed in this study, TRIPS is yet to be domesticated in Nigeria. To domesticate TRIPS, the Federal Ministries of Justice, Health and Trade & Investments should present a bill to the National Assembly requesting for its ratification and domestication. It could therefore be concluded that the Nigerian Pharmaceutical Industry lacks the legal backing and technological capability to exploit the opportunities offered by the TRIPS flexibilities.

CHAPTER THREE

RESEARCH AND DEVELOPMENT ACTIVITIES IN NIGERIA'S PHARMACEUTICAL INDUSTRY

RACHAEL A. AYO-LAWAL

Introduction

Research and Development (R&D) occupy a central position in the development of a vibrant, innovative and sustainable manufacturing pharmaceutical industry. Research has been considered to be a fundamental ingredient for action (Eisenberg, 2001), and is one of the most important activities of the pharmaceutical industry. Worldwide pharmaceutical R&D amounted to a total of US $141 billion in 2006, had an increase of 40% in 2015 and was projected to attain a growth of 60% in 2020 (Varntanian, 2018).

R&D activities are generally grouped into three types: basic, applied and experimental development. Basic research is primarily focused towards the creation of new knowledge or advancement of scientific knowledge, without any particular application or use in view. It is described as original experimental or theoretical work undertaken mainly to acquire new knowledge of the underlying foundation of phenomena and observable facts, without immediate commercial objectives or any particular application or use in view (Mansfield 1980; Frascati Manual 2002). Applied research is also conducted to acquire new knowledge, but it is directed towards a specific practical aim or objective to resolve an identified real-world problem (Driskell et al., 2014). Experimental development is directed towards producing new materials, products or devices, installing new processes, systems or services, or improving those already produced or installed.

This section discusses the status of, as well as issues surrounding R&D in Nigeria (both from schools of pharmacy and pharma firms) to support local pharmaceutical industry. First, we shall discuss results from the schools of pharmacy.

A. Status and Forms of Research & Development

i. Schools of Pharmacy

A total of 57 researchers from schools of pharmacy in Nigerian universities responded to the question on the form of research commonly conducted. The proportions of the researchers with respect to the form of research conducted are as indicated in Figure 3.1.

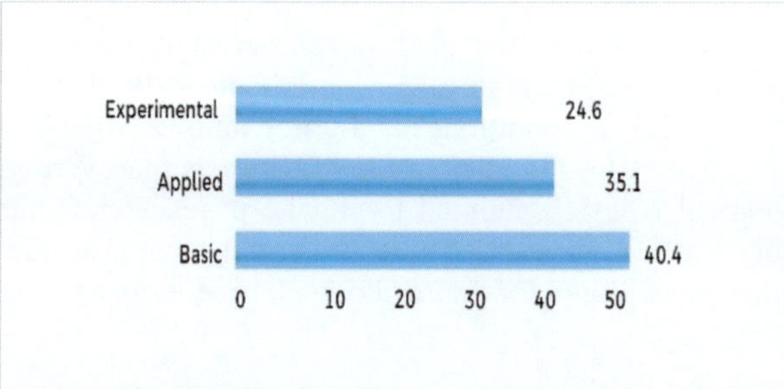

Figure 3.1: Types of Research Commonly Conducted among Researchers in Nigerian Schools of Pharmacy

This result revealed that basic research is conducted by the highest proportion of respondents. Although the impact on productivity of the different forms of research has been established, applied research and experimental development are more desirable for industrial (such as pharma) applications. It is worrisome to note that about 40% of the R&D undertaken by researchers in Nigerian schools of pharmacy is basic research, which may not be of immediate use in the pharma firms. This result agrees with the result of Musa (1988), where it was noted that the bulk of Nigerian university researchers are driven by demand for publications toward career advancement as against industrial application. However, about 35% of the research is applied, while about 25% is experimental development.

When Pharmaceutical R&D was inquired, approximately 65% (N=62) of the researchers attested to being involved in conducting drug development research activities (Figure 3.2).

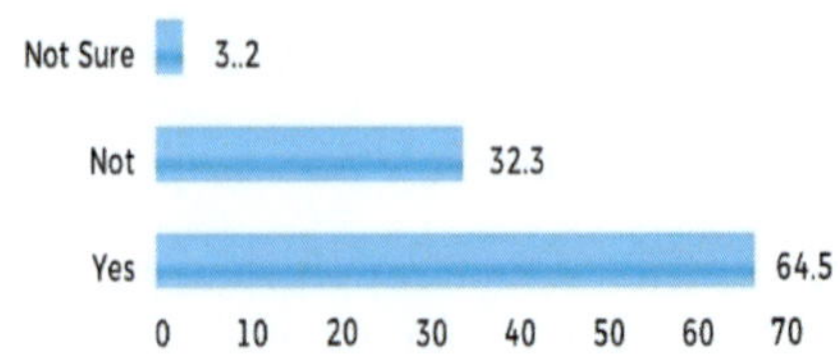

Figure 3.2: Researchers Involvement in Drug Development Studies

It is encouraging to know that drug development research towards the development of Active Pharmaceutical Ingredients (API) for medicines to address different disease conditions is on-going among Nigerian university pharma researchers. Close to 60% of the researchers that were involved in drug development research claimed to engage in researches aimed at the development of API (Figure 3.3). These API could become springboards for the launching of new drugs for the Nigerian pharma industry in the future.

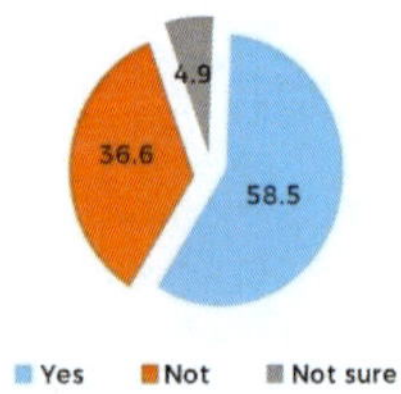

Figure 3.3: Researchers Involvement in APIs Development Research

The respondents who did not conduct research on API development refrained from doing so for several reasons presented in Figure 3.4. The most prominent of the reasons is a lack of funds to conduct the research (34.9%), followed by the non-availability of facilities/infrastructures (20.3%) and little/no institutional support (18.8%). Interestingly, about 10% of the respondents claimed that a lack of expertise prevented them from conducting API development research. This is a call for the refocusing of pharmaceutical training in Nigerian universities to adequately empower pharmacy graduates to enable them to conduct applied and experimental development researches.

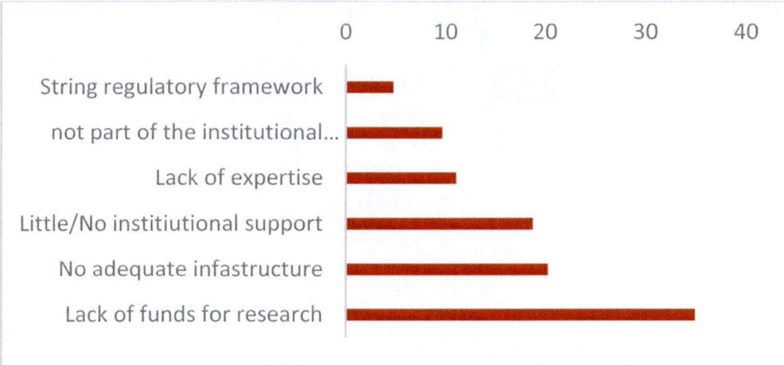

Figure 3.4: Reasons why Nigerian Schools of Pharmacy do not conduct API Researches (N=69)

Research leading to API development is capital-intensive, requiring sophisticated equipment which might not be readily available in many universities. The absence of such equipment is well documented. For instance, Yusuf (2012) reported that inadequate and irregular funding, and poor or obsolete research infrastructure, are among the factors impeding actualisation of high impact research in Nigeria. To corroborate this, the African Union (AU, 2015) attested that infrastructure, financial and knowledge resources are all among the prevailing challenges besetting investment in R&D in African nations. Consequently, research activities from universities do not translate into technological advancement for the country.

ii. Pharmaceutical Firms

Obviously, the existence of a functional R&D department in a pharma firm could be an indication of the firm's readiness to innovate. Among the 27 pharmaceutical firms that answered the question on the availability of an in-house R&D department, 13 (48.1%) answered in the affirmative (Figure 3.5). As expected, the commonest form of research undertaken by the firms with a functioning R&D department was drug/pharmaceutical research, which was conducted by 68.8% of respondents. About 28.1% of the firms claimed they conduct research on medicinal plants, while 21.9% and 28.1% claimed they conduct basic and market research respectively.

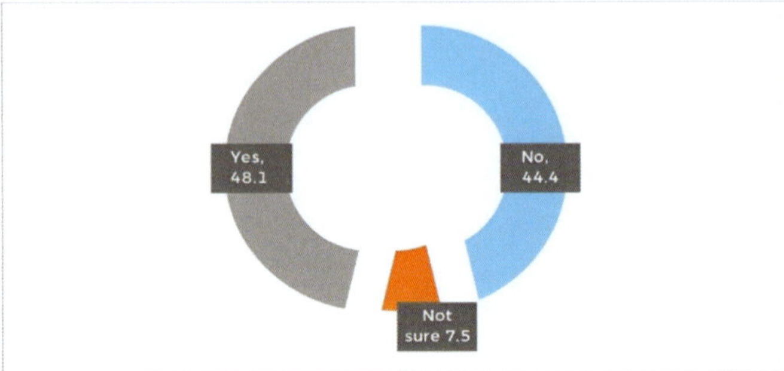

Figure 3.5: Availability of In-house R&D Department in Pharma Firms

B. Funding of R&D

i. Schools of Pharmacy

The level of awareness of the researchers on existing national, regional and international donor organisations that have an interest in funding pharmaceutical R&D are established in this study. Our results show that most of the researchers are not aware of funding opportunities at the three levels mentioned. Only 20.8% of the researchers are aware of funding agencies or organisations at the national level, 13.5% are aware of those at a regional level, while 37.1% are aware of funding agencies at the international level (Figure 3.6). According to Baro (2017) and Egwunyenga (2008), a good number of academic staff in Nigerian universities do not have access to research grants, for many reasons. The first of which is a lack of awareness, which agrees with the current findings. According to the two studies, many Nigerian lecturers opined that various calls for research grant proposals are not well advertised or publicised, but restricted in their circulation to a few researchers. To create better awareness of funding opportunities, the respondents suggested the use of institutional media such as radio, bulletins, and websites. However, the result of this study suggests that Nigerian pharmaceutical researchers are more conversant with international funding opportunities than national, local or regional ones, thereby suggesting either a shortage of, or a low level of funding opportunities from the latter sources.

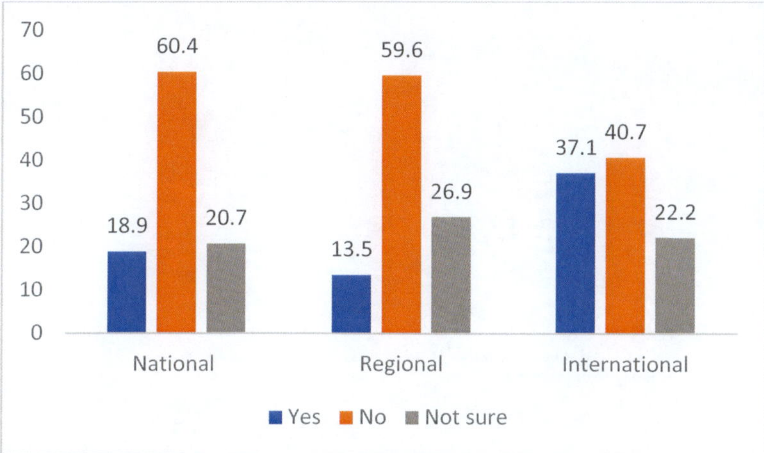

Figure 3.6: Awareness of Research Funding Opportunities Among Researchers in Nigerian Schools of Pharmacy (%)

Between the years 2015 and 2019, only 20.4, 12.5 and 25.0% of respondents accessed grants for pharma R&D from national, regional and international bodies respectively (Figure 3.7). These values are low and confirm the lack of awareness of funding opportunities among the respondents as earlier indicated by Figure 3.6. Grantsmanships among the academic staff in Nigerian universities have reportedly been poor. For instance, Bako (2005) and Baro et al. (2017) reported that only a few academic staff in the Nigerian higher education system have received grants for their research work. In addition to ignorance/lack of knowledge of funders, other reasons adduced to this poor access to grants include: sentiment/bias in the selection of proposal, sub-standard proposal, lack of motivation, bureaucracies involved, shortage of time to conduct research as a result of increasing staff/student ratio, and teaching or other pressing academic engagements (Bello 2012; Yusuf, 2012; Baro et al., 2017).

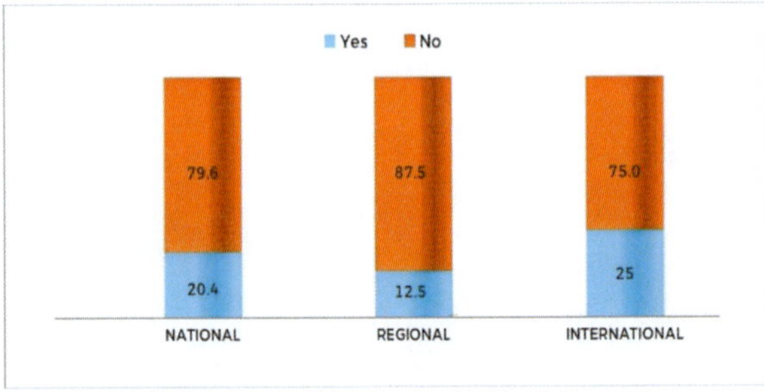

Figure 3.7: Levels of National, Regional and International Grants Obtained by Researchers of Nigerian Schools of Pharmacy

These results further revealed that fewer Nigerian pharma researchers received grants from national or local funders compared with those that received grants from international funders between 2015 and 2019. Most R&D in Africa is funded by the public sector, with significant proportions of financing in many countries emanating from international funders (Simpkin, 2019). This seems to be the case regarding pharma research in Nigeria. This situation is unlike that in the countries in the Organisation for Economic Co-operation and Development (OECD), where the largest source of R&D funds is the private sector. However, many challenges limit private sector involvement and investment in R&D in African countries; these include unstable political environments, poor governance and corruption (Geuna,1999; Donwa 2006; Simpkin 2019).

This study identified nine sources of funding for pharma R&D in Nigerian schools of pharmacy as displayed in Figure 3.8. Chief among these sources is funding from the individual researchers/self, as was indicated by 69.6% of the respondents. This result re-affirms the reports of the authors who have previously reported poor, low, and irregular funding of R&D activities in Nigeria; and reports that the highest volume of R&D funds comes from the income (mainly salaries) of academic staff members (Nworgu, 2006; Akpochafo, 2009; Akpan et al., 2010; Siyanbola et al., 2012; Baro, 2017). The results of this study show that this pattern of funding has not changed; rather there is an increase in the volume of self-sponsored research from an average of 17% that was reported by Siyanbola et al. (2012) to 57% among pharma researchers that were covered in this study. Self-sponsorship is closely followed by funding by the Tertiary Education Trust Fund (TETFUND), while university research grants were in the third position.

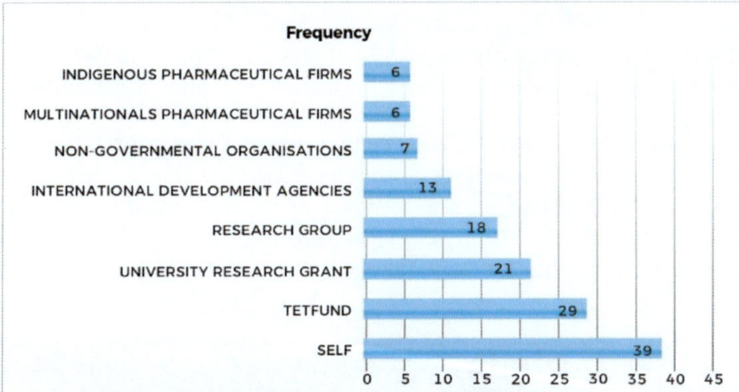

Figure 3.8: Sources of Funds for Pharma R&D Activities among Lecturers in Schools of Pharmacy

TETFUND was set up as an intervention fund to collect, manage and disburse Education Tax funds that are obtained from the private sector to government-owned tertiary education institutions in Nigeria. Over the years, the TETFUND has been funding R&D activities in Nigeria's tertiary institutions. Being the second highest source of pharmaceutical research funds in Nigeria accords with the findings of Baro (2017) who reported that TETFUND is the highest funding agency that academic staff members have received research grants from.

Apart from TETFUND, the respondents attested to receiving funds from the Federal Government of Nigeria (FGN) through other sources such as the Raw Materials Research and Development Council (RMRDC). Research grants from individual university also have impacts on the pharma R&D landscape in Nigeria. Again, Baro et al. (2017) reported that aside from TETFUND, researchers received an appreciable level of funding from the University of Ibadan Senate Grant. It therefore follows that sponsorship for pharma R&D in Nigerian universities is mainly from self, government and university research grants.

The study further reveals that the researchers received very low levels of grant from pharma firms (both indigenous and multinationals). This is a worrisome situation that indicates weak interactions between the duo regarding R&D activities.

Regional and international organisations that have given research grants to some of the respondents in the past are: Africa Research Exchange Funds, African Academy of Science, United Nations International Children's Emergency Fund (UNICEF), United Nations Industrial Development Organization (UNIDO), and the World Bank. There are several other organisations that the researchers could approach for pharma R&D funding in the future. They only have to search for them and apply as appropriate.

Table 3.1 presents the specific level of involvement/commitment of each of these categories of sources of funds to the researchers. The table shows that from 10 to 100% of R&D funding comes from the individual researcher/self among 39 respondents. The percentage contribution of TETFUND ranged from 3 to 80% for about 29 respondents.

Table 3.1: Contributions of Various Sources of Funds for Pharma R&D in Nigerian Universities

	Number of Respondents	Minimum	Maximum	Mean	Standard Deviation
Federal Government	9	0.0	20.0	5.1	6.9
International Development Agencies	13	0.0	100.0	19.0	28.1
TETFUND	29	3.0	80.0	30.3	25.5
University Research Grant	21	2.0	100.0	19.6	21.1
Multinationals	6	0.0	110.0	23.3	42.6
Indigenous Pharmaceutical Firms	6	0.0	30.0	10.3	10.6
NGOs	7	0.0	45.0	21.1	16.4
Research Group	18	0.0	100.0	39.1	32.2
Self	39	10.0	100.0	64.3	30.8

Source: Field Survey

Figure 3.9 presents information on recipients of grants from non-government organisations (NGOs). The figure revealed that 62 (29.0%) of pharma researchers that responded to the study have received research grants from NGOs in the past. This suggests a poor or low engagement/sponsorship of research by the NGOs. NGOs are private organizations that pursue activities to relieve suffering, promote the interests of the poor, protect the environment, provide basic social services, or undertake community development independent of the government

(Delisle et al., 2005). Two main distinct categories of NGOs according to purposes are: Economic development & infrastructure and Research.[1]

In research, NGOs play key roles especially in fiscal matters. This includes the provision of direct funding for projects, administration of research grants, identification and linking of potential funders (especially from the private sector) to a research group, or acting as a fiduciary agent for a grant to a research organization that is exploring an issue related to an NGO program (Delisle et al., 2005). The result (Figure 3.9) suggests that either health-aligned NGOs in Nigeria do not function in this regard or pharma researchers in Nigerian universities are yet to fully tap into the funding activities of these NGOs, both from local and international sources.

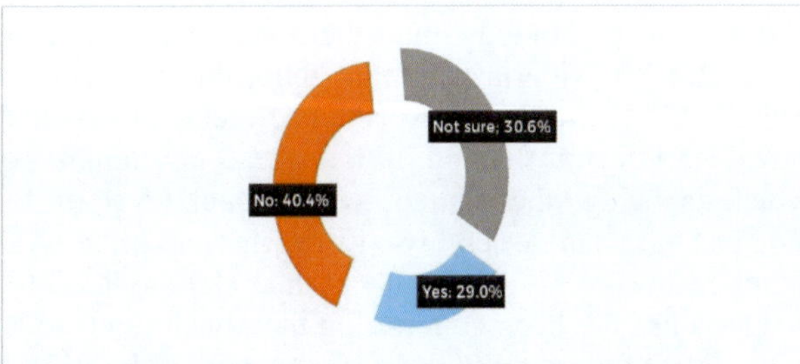

Figure 3.9: Accessing of R&D Grants from NGOs by Nigerian Pharmaceutical Researchers

Many reasons were given for the low funding of R&D with grants from NGOs among the Nigerian pharmaceutical researchers that responded to the survey. As presented in Figure 3.10, about 25% of the respondents claimed they were not aware of such opportunities, while about 29.0% claimed they were aware, but had yet to explore the opportunities. Other researchers who applied for such grants were either unsuccessful (19%) or did not receive any response from the NGOs. The NGOs that have funded the respondents' pharma research were UNIDO and International Foundation for Science.

[1] http://www.globalpolicy.org/ngos/role/intro/growth2000.htm

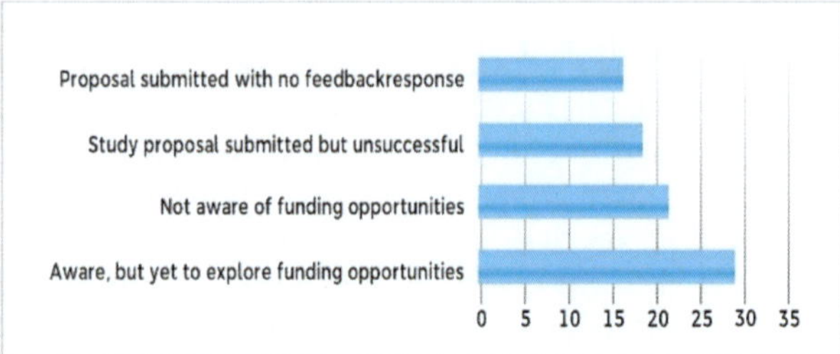

Figure 3.10: Reasons for Not Accessing R&D Funds from NGOs by Nigerian Pharmaceutical Researchers

From the above, it is obvious that the funds that are available for pharmaceutical R&D in Nigeria are small; hence the researchers are unable to conduct the R&D as would be expected of them. The poor funding of pharmaceutical R&D is a reflection of the overall low funding of R&D in Nigeria, which is below the agreed international level of funding for research. For instance, the Assembly of the African Union (AU) in 2007 urged its members to commit at least 1% of their GDP to R&D (AU, 2007). However, Nigeria has not been committing that much funds to R&D. Data from Nigeria's R&D Survey of 2006/2007 (NACETEM, 2011) shows that Nigeria's Gross Expenditure on Research and Development (GERD) was N45.9 billion; that is, US $583.2 million (2009).[2] As a share of the nation's GDP, this was only 0.2%, and is far below the 1% goal agreed by the AU.

ii. Pharmaceutical Firms

The present results found that pharma firms in Nigeria do not obtain R&D funding from external sources. All the 32 firms that participated in this study claimed that their R&D funds come solely from within the firm; that is, they are self-sponsored.

[2] 1 USD = 78.62 NGN in 2009 PPP

C. Challenges Confronting Nigerian Companies Intending to Start Local Production of API and Possible Solutions

Active Pharmaceutical Ingredients are compound(s) in a drug formulation that impart the desired therapeutic effect on them (Kaplan and Laing, 2005). Figure 3.11 shows that only three (9.7%) firms indicated they do some in-house production of API; out of these, two firms claimed they produce API for malaria drugs, while one (3.1%) indicated the product is targeted at the treatment of antacid.

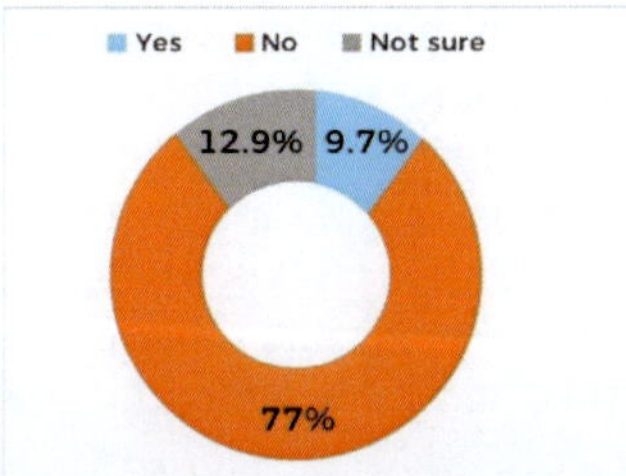

Figure 3.11: In-house Production of APIs by Nigerian Pharma Firms

From the key informant interviews with government and regulatory agencies (Federal Ministry of Health, NAFDAC, Pharmacists Council of Nigeria), it was gathered that no certification has hitherto been granted to any pharma firm to locally produce API of any drug in Nigeria, although some firms indicated they locally produce the ingredients for anti-malaria and antacid drugs as earlier mentioned. The claims of industrial production of anti-malaria and antacid drugs corroborate the report of Siyanbola et al. (2012), which stated that some Nigerian pharma firms make use of local raw materials for drug production. However, the disclosures of the NAFDAC and the Ministry of Health officials suggest that the use of such locally prepared API/concentrate, though efficacious, has not been approved by appropriate regulators in the industry. Notwithstanding that the development of API is an uphill task, about 60% of the university pharmaceutical researchers who responded to the study claimed to be involved in API development R&D (Figure 3.3).

In an interview conducted during the study, one of the key informants stated that:

> The production of API is a capital-intensive project that requires many things such as good infrastructure, political consciousness, and a well-designed programme to achieve it.

To start local production of API in Nigeria, therefore, the informant emphasized the need for a functional petrochemical industry, given that a lot of chemical inputs from that sector would be needed in the synthesis of API. In corroborating this, another key informant stated that Nigeria has, to some extent, got the needed capability and knowledge, but the petrochemical industry, which would provide about 60% of the synthetic materials needed for the development of the API, has to be established as well. The poor industrial base, particularly in the petrochemical industry, was mentioned by another key informant as one of the major challenges confronting the production of API in the country. The informant further reported that in other countries such as India and China, where generic medicines are manufactured, their governments play key roles through targeted research and innovation funds, venture funds and other entrepreneurship policies to increase local participation and attract foreign direct investments (FDIs) into the sector.

It was mentioned during the interview that NIPRD in the past proved its capability by extracting artemisinin from artemisia plants. This is the first stage of API development. However, R&D could provide industrial production processes for the production of API from synthetic materials derivable from petrochemical products. Industrial production of the API would ensure better sustainability of production as against the extraction of natural compounds from plants. Drug production from herbs is not sustainable and mass production of such drugs may be difficult. It was also revealed that NIPRD has conducted a background assessment of some medicines of high priority for the management of some diseases, and found that a sustainable source of the API for such medicines is synthetic petrochemical products. The Agency has since approached the Nigerian National Petroleum Corporation in this regard. Another ray of hope is the Dangote refinery which is under construction, which the Agency has equally approached for the possibility of supply of such products, once the refinery becomes operational.

In addition to the high capital outlay involved in the production of API, an informant also stressed other issues of importance including stable power, taxation, human capital, non-availability of raw materials, etc., as impediments to the local production of API.

The surveyed pharma firms rated their perception of the various factors impeding the local production of API, and their views are presented in Figure 3.12. The factors that the firms considered to have high impact include inadequate power supply, high capital outlay, WHO certification process, as well as intellectual property issues. The lack of incentives is considered by the majority to moderately affect the production of API.

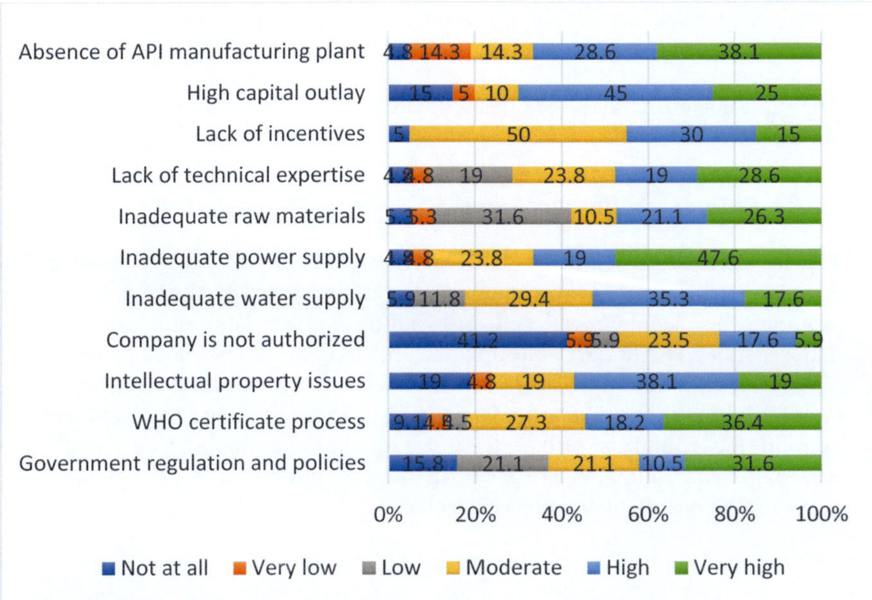

Figure 3.12: Pharma Firms' Perception of the Factors Affecting Production of API in Nigeria

D. On-going Activities of Knowledge Centres in Developing Locally Available Pharmaceutical Raw Materials to Support Their Industrial Usage

Given the current state of the Nigerian economy, the need for competitiveness, innovativeness and value-addition to the abundant natural resources cannot be overemphasised. Addition of value to local products with industrial utilisation would enhance their market value thereby promoting the local economy. To achieve this goal, the Nigerian government establish institutions (universities and research institutes), for knowledge generation. However, past efforts have not yielded much benefit, and most of the processed industrial raw materials used by local firms are still being imported, while the locally available ones remain in unprocessed raw forms. According to RMRDC (2016) Nigeria's potential for production of a wide range of raw materials needs revitalisation, with an appropriate stimulus targeted at commodity groups where the country has comparative and competitive advantages. Inadequate business infrastructure, including poor power supply, weak bureaucratic institutions and corruption, are among several factors that have negatively impacted on the existing potentials in the country.

The on-going R&D activities in the institutions visited during this survey are hereafter reported:

i. Raw Materials Research and Development Council (RMRDC)

The Raw Materials Research and Development Council (RMRDC) is an agency of the Federal Government of Nigeria vested with the mandate to promote the development and utilization of Nigeria's industrial raw materials. In 2016, as part of its mandate, the agency published the National Strategy for Competitiveness in Raw Materials and Products Development Plan for Nigeria. The plan articulates strategic issues in each sector that will help in the country's efforts toward reducing the importation of raw materials. The following are some of the recommended implementation plans for the chemical and pharma sector:

- Local production of API through partnership;
- Develop petrochemical industry to provide inputs for manufacture of items in the sector;
- Develop organic chemicals and pharmaceuticals from locally-available plant resources;
- Promote the procurement and patronage of the local pharmaceutical industry;
- Investment in local production of inputs such as adhesives, colorants, printing inks, etc.

Hitherto, the RMRDC has funded several researches on the development of local materials for use by the pharma firms with several breakthroughs/successes recorded. This was revealed during the key informant interview with a representative of the Pharmaceutical Material Division of the Council. The officer revealed that Nigerian pharma firms currently depend on importation of raw material for up to 80% of drugs manufactured in Nigeria; hence, the council is doing a lot to ensure that pharma raw materials are available locally for the firms to use. The officer however lamented that most multinational firms are not interested in using Nigerian local raw materials.

Major on-going activities targeted at the development of local pharmaceutical raw materials include the development of such products as: calcium carbonate, pharmaceutical grade starch, anti-diabetes nutraceutical, phytomedicine for the treatment of tuberculosis, and a material for the treatment of cardiovascular diseases. All these products have a high local content and they are in various stages of development. For instance, the anti-diabetes nutraceutical was at the stage of clinical trials at the time of this survey in 2019. The agency (in collaboration with NIPRD and SHETSCO) has also successfully developed pharmaceutical grade starch and has utilised same as the pharma excipient in the production of analgesic, and obtained standard products. The interviewee further stated that in the development of any useful product from research sponsored by the Council, a pilot plant is built to test-produce it, before such product is eventually commercialised.

Talking about what needs to be done to enhance the Council's efforts, the officer suggested that:

> there should be a government policy that would encourage the pharma firms to use local raw materials.

In addition, it was suggested that clusters should be formed for the development of pharmaceutical raw materials, especially those derived from domestic medicinal plants, to ensure sustainability in their production as pharmaceutical raw materials.

ii. Nigeria Natural Medicine Development Agency (NNMDA)

The Nigeria Natural Medicine Development agency is a public research institute that was established by the Federal Government of Nigeria in 1997. The core mandates of the Agency are to research, develop, document, preserve, conserve, commercialise and promote Nigeria's Natural Medicine (Traditional/Indigenous Healthcare Systems, medications and non-medications, healing arts, science and technology). The Agency is also expected to facilitate the integration of the Trado-Healthcare systems into the National Healthcare Delivery System. During an interview with an official of the Agency, it was revealed that they conduct research on various natural materials; this is followed by documentation of the outcome, publication of findings, and their commercialisation. These products are thereafter taken up by the private sector (natural or orthodox medicine) for production and eventual integration into Nigerian health care and management.

In addition, the Agency has facilitated the cultivation of medicinal plants on specialised farms, one in each geopolitical zone of the country. The purpose of this is to properly develop and cultivate identified medicinal plants in the areas where they grow best. The farms would also preserve the local knowledge base on the plants, preserve plants that are about to go into extinction, and facilitate the study and documentation of the biotic and abiotic factors and the general cultivation conditions needed for medicinal plants to be grown, domesticated, cultivated and conserved.[3] Products such as standardized extracts, nutraceuticals, health foods, dietary supplements, etc. can thereafter be develop from the local herbs.

Finally, the Agency is involved in the training of the practitioners who are involved in the cultivation of medicinal plants. These products could then form the basic raw materials for the pharma industry. It was also revealed that NNMDA has conducted comprehensive studies into indigenous Nigerian natural medicine, both in terms of knowledge and practice, and NAFDAC had certified some of the products that resulted from the R&D activities. Various herbal therapies and nutritional supplements directed at the following health challenges have been successfully developed by NNMDA: diabetes, arthritis, topical dermatitis (cream, ointments, soap), erectile dysfunction, prostate enlargement, cosmetic and beauty products, neglected tropical diseases (herbal mullocides), and natural products for the treatment of livestock diseases.

iii. The National Institute for Pharmaceutical Research and Development (NIPRD)

The National Institute for Pharmaceutical Research and Development (NIPRD) is a public research institute that was established by a Federal Government of Nigeria order in 1989. Its vision is "to be a Centre of Excellence in research and development of phytomedicines, pharmaceutical and biological products, drugs and diagnostics towards improving the health and well-being of mankind". More specifically, the agency was established to undertake R&D activities on drugs, biological products including

[3] http://nnmda.gov.ng/development-of-mapps/

vaccines, and pharmaceutical raw materials from indigenous natural resources, using appropriate science and technology methodologies.[4]

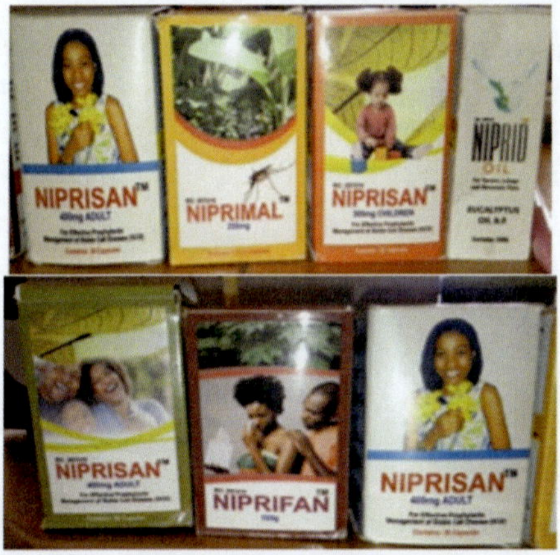

Figure 3.13: Some Pharmaceutical Products Successfully Developed by NIPRD

According to the informant from the agency, the Institute has carried out substantial R&D for product and process development with relevance to drug-related products, in line with its mandate (Figure 3.13). Six key products have been successfully developed while about 22 are ongoing and nearing completion. One of the flagship products is Niprisan/Nicosan that is used for the management of sickle cell anaemia. The product was granted orphan drug status by both the United States Food and Drug Administration and the European Medicine Evaluation Agency. The fact that Niprisan/Nicosan was the only therapy that is available for the management of sickle cell anaemia, which affects over 10 million patients in sub-Saharan Africa, gave a boost to the local pharmaceutical industry. NIPRD is presently developing other phytomedicines for the management of prevailing diseases. These include:

- NIPRIMAL - Treatment of malaria;
- NIPRID OIL - A eucalyptus product from natural sources for the treatment of catarrh and cough;
- NIPRIFAN - Treatment of fungal diseases;
- NIPRIMUNE - An immune booster. The product has successfully undergone clinical trial up to phase II;
- NANOMET: An antidiabetic;

[4] http://www.niprd.gov.ng/about-us/

- NIPRIBOIL: A cocktail of agents from medicinal plants with antiviral activities specifically formulated for the cure/treatment of the Ebola virus.

Furthermore, NIPRD in association with RMRDC and SHESTCO has developed the production of pharmaceutical grade starch from non-food sources like weed (Tacca). The institute has also established collaboration with many pharma firms in the area of product and staff development among others.

CHAPTER FOUR

INTELLECTUAL PROPERTY RIGHTS, TECHNOLOGY TRANSFER AND WHO CERTIFICATION

CALEB M. ADELOWO

Introduction

The pharmaceutical manufacturing sector is a knowledge-intensive sector that requires substantial investment in research and development (R&D). It also requires continuous training or capacity development of staff for the development of new medicines and the refinement of existing ones. Most of these R&D and training efforts are targeted at identifying and creating new chemical entities or active pharmaceutical ingredients to address existing or new disease conditions. The development of these medicines involves huge capital outlay by pharmaceutical manufacturing companies on equipment and the remuneration of researchers. Consequently, the medicines that are developed from these research efforts are the intellectual property of their developers and are protected with patents. Patents are granted to individuals or organisations whose inventions meet the criteria of novelty, non-obviousness and industrial applicability. The basic aims of the patent are to prevent unauthorised use of the inventions and to provide incentives for the inventors to recoup their investment over a number of years, usually 20 years (WIPO, 2004). When a patent is granted for a new medicine, the owner is bestowed the exclusive right to make commercial production of the medicine. In exercising the right, the patent holder may grant one or more companies licenses to manufacture the medicine for the payment of some royalties.

As much as the rights of the creators and investors are well protected, the issues of public health and rights to essential medicines are also protected and should not be in jeopardy. Given the huge financial and technological investments required to develop and produce medicines, some of the strategies adopted in some climes to develop a pharma sector include tax rebates, targeted procurement policies, an efficient intellectual property system and technology transfer policies. The latter is a key factor for attracting FDIs and technical assistance/support to the sector. A number of best practices have shown that technical collaboration with foreign investors in whatever form is a key driver in the pharmaceutical sector. For instance, in 2018, one of the pharma firms in Nigeria took important steps by unveiling a new oxytocin injection for pregnant women through collaborative efforts with the United States Pharmacopeia.[1]

In this section, the focus is on how pharmaceutical firms in Nigeria address intellectual property issues, particularly as they affect antiretrovirals (ARVs), malarial and other generic medicines in the country. Although the majority of the pharma firms in the country do not have the capability to produce API, they do have the capacity to formulate, mix, package and market the drugs. Most of the API are imported from China, India, Pakistan and other Asian countries, while a few come from the West: Europe and North America. Most of the imported API are for generic drugs, which are variants of the originals that are patented; and because their processes of development have required less R&D than those of the original, they are usually cheaper than the originals. Even in the advanced countries, many people still prefer generic drugs because patented drugs are usually more expensive. During the 2020 pandemic, the generic hydroxychloroquine (HCQ) used in fighting COVID-19 in the USA and other parts of the world was manufactured in India, while the API for it were in turn sourced from China (Privali, 2020). It is therefore important for Nigeria to build a strong industrial base for the manufacture of API.

The results of the field survey in respect of production of ARVs are presented in Table 4.1, which showed that about 80% of the pharma firms in Nigeria do not manufacture ARVs. This has resulted in a huge reliance on importation of the drug into Nigeria. The two firms that claimed they are producing ARVs in the country are Fidson Ltd. and May & Baker Ltd, representing 8% of the sampled pharma firms. One other firm claimed that it developed the formulas for production in-house. On the production of generic medicines, about 32% of the firms responded affirmatively, while a larger percentage (36.4%) were not involved in the production of generic drugs. The kind of production agreement entered into by the firms that

[1] Anudu, O. "Nigerian pharmaceutical industry: Big steps, setbacks, prospects" Bussinessday newspaper, July 2019. Available at: https://businessday.ng/real-sector/article/nigerian-pharmaceutical-industry-big-steps-setbacks-prospects/

produce the drugs includes franchising by three (9.4%), voluntary licensing by two (6.3%) and compulsory licensing by one (3.1%). The results suggest that most of these firms are not into drug production from raw materials, but engage in mixing, formulating and packaging, particularly for ARVs and other generic drugs.

Table 4.1: Types of Drugs Produced and Nature of Production Agreement with Intellectual Property Owners for antiretrovirals (ARVs) and other generic medicines

Does your firm produce ARVs? (N=25)	Frequency	%
No	20	80.0
Not sure	3	12.0
Yes	2	8.0
Does the firm produce other generic medicines? (N=22)		
No	8	36.4
Not sure	7	31.8
Yes	7	31.8
Nature of production Agreements (N=5) *		
Franchising	3	9.4
Licensing	2	6.3
Compulsory License	1	3.1

Source: Field Survey
*Multiple response

The possession of intellectual property (IP) for drug production is strategic to the positioning of a company for competition and the extent of security it offers during major disease outbreaks. Pharma firms in advanced and emerging economies generate IP through apt investment in R&D or licensing. In Nigeria, very few pharma firms have invested in R&D, but all rely on one or other form of IP sourcing. Table 4.2 shows the sources of IPs being used by the 13 firms that responded to this question. The results from the field survey showed that 9.4% of the pharma firms obtained IP through voluntary licensing and from local universities, 6.3% obtain them from research institutes, private research organisation and donor agencies, while 3.1% obtain the IP from foreign universities.

Table 4.2: Sources of Intellectual Property Used for Production by Pharma Firms

Intellectual Property Sources	Frequency	%
Voluntary License	3	9.3
Local Universities	3	9.3
Research Institutes	2	6.4
Private Research Organisation	2	6.4
Donor Agencies	2	6.4
Foreign Universities	1	3.1
Compulsory License	0	0
Public Domain	0	0
Diaspora	0	0

Source: Field Survey

Compulsory license has to do with the application of the Trade Related aspect of Intellectual Properties' (TRIPS)[2] flexibilities in gaining access to essential medicines, though the TRIPS agreement is yet to be domesticated in Nigeria. Therefore, the application of TRIPS flexibilities in the country as claimed by one of the firms is uncertain but not impossible. The limited number of responses from pharma firms on their level of compliance with the government directives on TRIPS flexibilities could be a direct indication of poor awareness or understanding of the matter by the firms. Out of the 17 pharma firms that claimed to comply with compulsory licensing, 52.9% of them claimed to comply very much, while only 5.9% of them had very little compliance. On the exhaustion regime, about 33.3% each of the pharma firms complied much and very much, while 16.7% of them had little and very little compliance levels. The levels of compliance with government use as claimed by the firms were very much (28.6%), much (50%), little (14.3%) and very little (7.1%). There is also high level of compliance with research exemption, as the majority of the firms claimed much compliance (66.7%) and very much compliance (8.3%). However, the levels of compliance with early working condition and data exclusivity are quite small, as shown in Table 4.3. These results are a clear indication of poor research activities among the pharma firms in the country. They also suggest that the sector depends largely on importation of key production inputs, especially API and manufacturing plants as noted by Wakeel and Ekundayo, (2016).

[2] Nigeria is a signatory to the Trade Related aspect of Intellectual Properties (TRIPS). Its flexibilities include the opportunity granted to each member state to define patentable subject matter and apply national peculiarities in the interpretation of the provisions of the treaty.

Table 4.3: Level of Compliance with Government Directives on TRIPS Flexibilities

Areas of TRIPS Flexibilities	Very much	Much	Little	Very Little	Not at all
Compulsory license (17)	52.9	41.2	0	5.9	0
Exhaustion regime (12)	33.3	33.3	16.7	16.7	0
Government use (14)	28.6	50.0	14 .3	7.1	0
Research exemption (12)	8.3	66.7	16.7	8.3	0
Early working condition (13)	7.7	30.8	38.5	23.1	0
Data exclusivity (14)	14.3	35.7	14.3	35.7	0

Source: Field Survey

On the question of WHO pre-qualification, the majority (64%) of the pharma firms have not acquired pre-qualification, stating that it requires high standards and a huge financial commitment (Table 4.4). The results further showed that 16% of the pharma firms have attained WHO pre-qualification status. Of these latter firms, 75% reported that they secured the pre-qualification through collaboration with other big pharma firms. The nature of their agreement with the bigger firms includes voluntary (33.3%) and restricted (66.7%) licensing. These results also suggest some deficiencies in the Nigerian pharma sector, where only a few pharma firms have licenses to manufacture under WHO pre-qualifications; albeit many of them under restricted licenses. A restricted license ties the licensee to the apron of licensor, indicating that most of the activities in the sector are dictated by foreign technological forces: the Nigerian government through the Ministry of Health merely provides regulatory and policy environments for the industry players.

Table 4.4: Position of Pharma Firms on WHO Pre-Qualification for Manufacturing of Medicine

The Firm Received WHO Pre-Qualification for the drugs it manufactures (N=25)	Frequency	%
No	16	64.0
Not sure	5	20.0
Yes	4	16.0
The Firm collaborated with Big Pharmaceutical Firms to Secure the Pre-Qualification (N=22)	**Frequency**	**%**
No	15	68.2
Not sure	4	18.2
Yes	3	13.6
Nature of the Agreement with Big Pharmaceutical Firms (N=3)	**Frequency**	**%**
Voluntary licensing	1	33.3
Restricted licensing	2	66.7

Source: Field Survey

On the number of WHO pre-qualified drugs produced by the pharma firms, just two firms reported that they manufacture ten generic medicines each, largely in the areas of malaria and other diseases (Table 4.5). As expected, no company among Nigerian pharmaceutical manufacturers is producing pre-qualified API and brand name medicines.

As earlier stated, WHO pre-qualification requires a huge financial commitment by any firm that intends to obtain the certification, though it would pay off on the long run. This made many Nigerian pharmaceutical manufacturers hold back from venturing into it. Reports from a key informant interview session revealed that a pharma firm made a huge investment to acquire WHO-prequalification, but after a while the company folded up for lack of patronage for its products.

Table 4.5: Number of Pre-Qualified Drugs Produced by Nigerian Pharma Firms

Prequalified Drugs	Number
Generic medicines	2
Brand Name	2
APIs	2
Disease Areas	**Number**
HIV/AIDS	0
Malaria	1
Others	1

Source: Field Survey

The Federal Government of Nigeria established some regulatory agencies including the National Agency for Food and Drug Administration and Control (NAFDAC), Standards Organisation of Nigeria (SON) and Pharmacists Council of Nigeria (PCN), whose activities cover the pharma sector among others. These agencies perform the specific function of guaranteeing smooth operation and healthy rivalry among the players. NAFDAC regulates and controls food and drugs administration in the country and ensures they meet specified safety levels; SON ensures that the equipment and machinery deployed in the sector measure up to the expected standards; while PCN provides guidelines to ensure that competent hands are engaged in pharmaceutical practices and also ensures that pharma premises across the country meet required standards.

Drugs and premises certification are also conducted by NAFDAC before the firms are allowed to commence operations, while drug certification is done for the drugs to be produced by the firms. About 87.1% of the firms claimed that all drugs they are producing are certified and approved by NAFDAC; while a few firms (12.9%) claimed that some of their drugs were approved. 18 firms responded to the question on meeting the standard requirements for production equipment. All the equipment was approved for 8 (44%) of the firms, only some of the equipment was approved for the same number of firms, while the persons that responded for 2 (11.1%) firms were not sure of the approval. Most of the firms (52.4%) also had the approval of the PCN to operate. (Table 4.6).

Table 4.6: Approvals Obtained by Pharma Firms for Medicines, Machinery and Premises

Regulatory Agencies	Yes, all	Yes, some	Not sure	Not at all
NAFDAC (N=31)	87.1	12.9	0	0
SON (N=18)	44.4	44.4	11.1	0
PCN (N=21)	52.4	38.1	9.5	0
PSN (N=18)	27.8	44.4	27.8	0

Source: Field Survey

Given the sensitivity of the sector to the human and economic potential of the country, it is very clear from the results of the analysis that the government gives priority to adequate regulation of pharmaceutical production, to deter unwholesome practices in the sector.

CHAPTER FIVE

INTERACTION WITHIN NIGERIA'S PHARMACEUTICAL INDUSTRY

ADESINA AYOBAMI OYEWALE

Introduction

The system of innovation in the pharmaceutical industry is characterized by high dependence on research and development (R&D) activities for either production of new drugs or improvement of existing ones. The R&D activities can be conducted in-house, in the laboratories of the industrial firms, or obtained from external sources such as universities, research institutes and patent documents. Even when a firm has a functioning in-house laboratory, to enable it to resolve problems and acquire new knowledge quickly, the firms may still depend on external sources.

All the 32 firms that responded to the study claimed they are aware of the Nigerian universities and research institutes which conduct R&D activities on drugs that are of interest to them. In confirming the claims, the firms indicated the names of the institutions. However, only six (30%) of the 20 firms that responded to a question on collaborating with universities claimed to do so; nine (45%) did not, while officials that responded for five firms (25%) were not sure. In addition, seven (35%) of those 20 firms also claimed to collaborate with research institutes, 11 (55%) did not, while two (10%) were not sure. Another possible source of knowledge for the development of new medicines is the indigenous herbal stock. Only 15 firms responded to the question on this source. Two (13.3%) of the firms claimed to collaborate with producers of indigenous herbal medicine, eight (53.3%) did not, while five (33.3%) were not sure.

In all, 31 of the firms stated different reasons for not collaborating with the institutions. The reason given by 22 (71%) firms was that the researchers are difficult to locate and, when they are found, the behaviours of the researchers make it appear that the problem cannot be solved in Nigeria.

Other reasons include a lack of opportunities, non-conducive environment within the institutions, unawareness of research areas and irregular university school calendar. Firms also indicated that the high costs of consultation and sustainability of such collaborations made them refrain from doing so. While one company claims it is looking forward to collaborating with the institutions, another claimed the collaborations it did in the past did not yield positive results. However, one firm expects researchers to approach it to initiate collaboration, possibly to showcase their abilities.

The firms that claimed to have collaborations with the institutions gave the strengths of their collaborations with the institutions on 12 areas of interest to the study. The responses of the firms are presented in Table 5.1.

A summary of the Table is that 11.3% of the pharmaceutical firms experienced very weak, weak or strong collaborations with research organisations, 28.2% experienced strong collaborations, while 37.9% experienced moderate collaborations. The above information implies that about 77.4% of the firms enjoyed at least moderately strong collaborations with the institutions in the 12 aspects of research-industry collaboration that were considered. If the "strength" of collaboration of the firms with research institutions could be equated with the "benefits" the firms obtained from such collaborations, it could be concluded that collaborating with the institutions had been beneficial to the industrial firms. Obviously, those firms that do not involve in collaborative activities are losing out on several beneficial issues, but unfortunately, many of them may not realise that. This ignorance keeps the firms from collaborating with the institutions that could be their source of help, thereby corroborating the view of Stankiewicz (1986), who remarked that the problem with ignorance is that it tends to be self-reinforcing; a firm that does not believe that it can gain anything by interacting with universities will refrain from doing so, thereby remaining ignorant.

The low level of interaction between Nigerian industrial firms and research organisations was reported by Oyewale (2010), who compared the interactions of university researchers with industrial firms in the Cocoa Processing, Pharmaceutical and Steel Manufacturing industries. The author revealed that interactions of the researchers from the three fields with industrial firms by means of Information/Knowledge exchange, Materials/Equipment usage and Finance were low. However, among the three, interactions involving Materials/Equipment usage were reported as the most prominent, followed by Information/Knowledge exchange, while interactions involving Finance were the least.

Table 5.1: Strengths of Collaborations of Nigerian Pharmaceutical Firms with Research Institutions

S/No	Object of Collaboration	Strength of Collaboration I	II	III	IV	V
1	Knowledge Sharing/Acquisition (N=12)	1 (8.3%)	0 (0%)	3 (25%)	6 (50%)	2 (16.7%)
2	Provision of R&D Facilities (N=12)	1 (3.1%)	0 (0%)	5 (15.6%)	4 (12.5%)	2 (6.3%)
3	Access to Laboratory Facilities (N=13)	1 (3.1%)	0 (0%)	4 (12.5%)	7 (21.9%)	1 (3.1%)
4	Staff Exchange with Research Institutions (N=10)	1 (3.1%)	2 (6.3%)	5 (15.5%)	0 (0%)	2 (6.3%)
5	Sponsorship for Fellowship Programmes (N=10)	2 (6.3%)	1 (3.1%)	5 (15.6%)	0 (0%)	2 (6.3%)
6	Endowment of Prizes (N=9)	1 (3.1%)	3 (9.4%)	4 (12.5%)	0 (0%)	1 (3.1%)
7	Endowment of Professorial Chairs (N=9)	1 (3.1%)	1 (3.1%)	6 (18.8%)	1 (3.1%)	0 (0%)
8	Provision of Research Grant (N=9)	2 (6.3%)	1 (3.1%)	1 (3.1%)	4 (12.5%)	1 (3.1%)
9	Granting of Internship (N=10)	1 (3.1%)	0 (0%)	5 (15.5%)	4 (12.5%)	0 (0%)
10	Industrial Attachment Programme (N=11)	2 (3.1%)	1 (0%)	5 (15.6%)	3 (9.4%)	2 (6.3%)
11	Sponsorship to Conference (N=9)	1 (3.1%)	3 (9.4%)	1 (3.1%)	3 (9.4%)	1 (3.1%)
12	Joint R&D Activities (N=10)	1 (6.3%)	3 (9.4%)	3 (9.4%)	3 (9.4%)	0 (0%)

Source: Field Survey

Key **I very Weak II. Weak .III. Moderate IV. Strong V. Very Strong**

The Nigerian government is aware of the poor linkages between knowledge centres (universities & research institutes) and industry. For instance, the Nigeria Industrial Revolution Plan (NIRP, 2014) mentioned inadequate interaction between academia, industry and government as one of the challenges in Nigeria, stating that it is inadequate, or in many cases lacking. Consequently, Nigeria has not been able to develop its own technology-niche from the group of proven and tested technologies developed in the country. The document further stated that the Nigerian government has historically not adequately facilitated interactions between industry, academia, and the public sector. This is possibly explained by the absence of an explicit policy statement or directive on linkages and interactions between the knowledge centres and industry in both the National Policy on Education and the Industrial Policy.

To address this lapse, the national Science, Technology and Innovation (STI) Policy (FMST, 2011) introduced the promotion of effective interactions, linkages and collaborations among the government, knowledge institutions and industries in all sectors including the health sector. The policy also provided for the strengthening of demand-driven R&D in natural and orthodox medicines and identified pharmaceutical research among the R&D policy strategies to be used in Health Research and Innovation. In addition, fostering interactions among universities, higher education and research institutions, industries and investors to generate innovations is included as a policy strategy for Industrial Research, Development and Production.

13 (40.6%) of the firms indicated that their joint R&D activities with research organisations are directed towards malaria, while one firm (3.1%) directed such research at HIV-AIDS. The collaborative R&D research resulted in new products for 10 (31%) firms, new processes for drug production for 5 (16%) firms and product enhancement/improvement for five (16%) of the firms. In addition, eight (25%) firms claimed they collaborate with other pharmaceutical firms, and such collaborations were mainly for capacity building and contract manufacturing.

An important factor that can encourage industrial firms to interact with knowledge centres is possession of in-house R&D facilities. Such facilities could encourage interactions between researchers of the firms and the knowledge centres. Researchers of industrial laboratories could form informal networks with researchers at universities or research institutes working in the same or complementary fields, to assist each other to resolve problems. Because of the cost involved, firms may be unable to employ the full spectrum of staff needed to run R&D laboratories; but the informal networks that are formed by their researchers with those from the knowledge centres could fill the gap. In support of this assertion, Malecki and Toole (1996) hint that networks could provide external sources of inputs that complement or substitute for the firm's internal capabilities.

R&D facilities are very expensive to establish and operate. However, UNCTAD (2009) reveals that Nigeria's government has several fiscal incentives to encourage firms to invest in R&D. Such provisions include the setting aside of up to 10% of their profits as reserves for R&D expenses; expenditure on commercialisation of R&D outputs that qualifies firms for a 20% investment tax credit; and corporate contributions to R&D carried out by universities and research institutes that are tax deductible, up to a maximum of 10% of profits. The document further claimed that draft legislation that was prepared in 2005 proposed to raise this cap to 15% of profits or 25% of the tax bill. As earlier reported, 13 (40.6%) of the firms claimed they have functioning in-house R&D departments.

Interactions by Knowledge Institutions

A total of 69 respondents from Faculties of Pharmacy in Nigerian universities responded to the study. From their responses, it was revealed that researchers of the faculties conduct researches whose outputs are useful to pharmaceutical industrial firms. Such researches include the development of anti-microbial agents, antibiotic medicines from leaf extracts, drug development from natural sources including herbal medicine, isolation of active anticancer agents, development of aphrodisiac drugs and formulations for anti-malaria drugs.

15 (22%) of the respondents indicated that researchers of their faculties collaborate with pharmaceutical industrial firms, 35 (51%) indicate the researchers do not, 13 (19%) claimed they were not sure, while 6 (9%) gave no response.

In the process of collaborating with pharmaceutical industrial firms, ten (14.5%) researchers shared knowledge with the firms, seven (10.1%) provided R&D services, ten (14.5%) provided laboratory facilities, three (4.3%) were involved in staff exchange, while two (2.9%) were involved in the training of industrial staff. In addition, eight (11.6%) researchers had received endowment prizes from the firms, seven (10.1%) had been awarded professorial chairs, five (7.2%) received research grants, seven (10.1%) enjoyed internship, while three (4.3%) had been involved in fellowship programmes with the firms. Other kinds of collaboration, where the respondents had been involved with industrial firms, were: student industrial attachment programme (12; 17.4%), sponsorship to conferences (8; 11.6%), joint R&D activities (4; 5.8%), funding of projects (5; 7.2%), research consultancy (5; 7.2%), use of firms' facilities (7; 10.1%), and contract research (2; 2.9%).

The strengths of the collaborations of the institutions and researchers as perceived by the lecturers for 16 areas of interest to the study are presented in Table 5.2.

In summary, 36.8% of the respondents rated the collaborations of pharmaceutical researchers with pharmaceutical firms as being very weak, while 30.8% rated them to be weak. In addition, about 18.9% respondents rated the collaborations to be moderate, 10.3% rated them to be strong, while 3.2% rated them to be very strong. These ratings imply that on average, about 32.4% of the researchers rated research-industry collaborations on the 16 aspects that were considered to be at least moderately strong, while close to 70% viewed the collaborations to be at least weak. The implication is that the researchers do not enjoy the benefits they expect from industrial firms.

Eight (21.6%) of the respondents of the Faculties of Pharmacy, in confirmation of collaborations of their faculties with industrial firms, indicated the names of industrial firms that they had collaborated with in the past. Two (2.9%) mentioned the research outputs that are being used by industrial firms as antimicrobial agents and microbial sensitivity disks. Six (8.7%) of the researchers indicated that researchers of their departments/faculties received commissioned research funds from industrial firms, while 47 (68.1%) did not. However, six (8.7%) were not sure.

The academics indicated the channels through which researchers of their departments/faculties disseminate research outputs to the public. 56 (81.2%) of the researchers indicated that the research outputs were disseminated through journal articles; 21 (30.4%) through books; 22 (31.9%) through technical reports; eight (11.6%) through monographs; four (5.8%) through policy briefs; three (4.3%) through white papers; and four (5.8) through working papers.

Six (8.7%) of the researchers indicated that researchers of their departments/faculties had received requests from pharmaceutical firms to conduct research on specific issues in the past, while 41 (59.4%) had not. However, 14 (20.3%) were not sure of such requests.

Table 5.2: Strengths of Collaborations of Nigerian Research Institutions with Pharmaceutical Firms

S/No	Object of Collaboration	Strength of Collaboration I	II	III	IV	V	Number of Firms
1	Knowledge Sharing	4 (28.6%)	3 (21.4%)	4 (28.6%)	3 (21.4%)	0 (0%)	14 (100%)
2	Provision of R&D Services/Facilities	4 (30.8%)	5 (38.5%)	2 (15.4%)	2 (15.4%)	0 (0%)	13 (100%)
3	Access to Laboratory Facilities	3 (20%)	5 (33.3%)	2 (13.3%)	4 (26.7%)	1 (6.7%)	15 (100%)
4	Staff Exchange with Industrial firms	3 (30%)	6 (60%)	1 (10%)	0 (0%)	0 (0%)	10 (100%)
5	Acceptance for Fellowship Programmes	4 (40%)	5 (50%)	1 (10.6%)	0 (0%)	0 (0%)	10 (100%)
6	Endowment of Prizes	5 (41.7%)	3 (25%)	1 (8.3%)	1 (8.3%)	2 (16.7%)	12 (100%)
7	Endowment of Professorial Chairs	5 (50%)	2 (20%)	2 (20%)	1 (10%)	0 (0%)	10 (100%)
8	Provision of Research Grant	5 (38.5%)	2 (15.4%)	4 (30.8%)	2 (15.4%)	0 (0%)	13 (100%)
9	Students' Industrial Attachment Programme	2 (13.3%)	1 (13.3%)	1 (46.7%)	4 (13.3%)	1 (13.3%)	1 (100%)
10	Sponsorship to Conference	4 (33.3%)	5 (41.7%)	2 (16.7%)	1 (8.3%)	0 (0%)	12 (100%)
11	Joint R&D Activities	6 (60%)	2 (20%)	2 (20%)	0 (0%)	0 (0%)	12 (100%)
12	Training of Staff	6 (50%)	3 (25%)	2 (16.7%)	1 (8.3%)	0 (0%)	12 (100%)
13	Funding of Projects	4 (44.4%)	4 (44.4%)	1 (11.1%)	0 (0%)	0 (0%)	9 (100%)
14	Research Consultancy	4 (33.3%)	4 (33.3%)	3 (25%)	1 (8.3%)	0 (0%)	12 (100%)
15	Use of Firm's Facilities	4 (40%)	3 (00%)	1 (10%)	1 (10%)	1 (10%)	10 (100%)
16	Contract Research	5 (62.5%)	3 (37.5%)	0 (0%)	0 (0%)	0 (0%)	8 (100%)

Source: Field Survey

Key **I** Very Weak **II.** Weak **.III.** Moderate **IV.** Strong **V.** Very Strong

Agency/Institution Based Interactions

The Pharmaceutical Society of Nigeria (PSN)

In its operation, the Pharmaceutical Society of Nigeria (PSN) relates with local pharmaceutical organisations such as the Nigerian Association of Pharmacists, and foreign ones like the Royal Pharmaceutical Society of Great Britain, pharmaceutical societies in the Americas, and Nigerian pharmacists in the diaspora. The PSN enhances information sharing by exchanging ideas and information related to pharmaceutical practice with these organisations. It also releases information obtained from outside to all members with a view to updating their knowledge to enable them to provide globally competitive services. The PSN is involved in advocacy to persuade government to enact policies that will promote the local pharmaceutical industry. The society is also involved in promoting R&D in Nigerian universities and gives scholarships and awards to brilliant students.

PSN has entered into agreements with the National Association of Pharmacists in Academia (NAPA) and the National Association of Industrial Pharmacists to develop substrates from local raw materials for use in manufacturing in order to replace imported ones. This is a deletion program, whereby some items such as pharmaceutical grade starch, colorant, and adjuvant excipients would no longer be imported within some years, thereby increasing the contribution of local content to total manufacturing. The Association is working with industry to provide funds to academics to conduct R&D in order to ensure that Nigeria starts to produce API, because it is an area where Nigeria is falling short. Therefore, a master plan and business feasibility study has been drawn up, while funding is being sought for the endeavour.

The Nigerian Natural Medicine Development Agency (NNMDA)

The Nigerian Natural Medicine Development Agency (NNMDA) has the mandate of researching, collecting documenting, publishing and training Nigerian Natural Medicine Practitioners and disseminating knowledge on natural indigenous medicine to the general public. NNMDA also has the mandate to conduct and commercialize its R&D products. In the discharge of these mandates, the Agency has developed several products to combat different aliments and is collaborating with pharmaceutical industrial firms for up-scaling of the R&D results. Presently, three pharmaceutical firms in Nigeria have shown interest in such products. The Agency is also developing raw materials for the pharmaceutical industry for both natural and orthodox medicinal practices. NNMDA is collaborating with some Nigerian universities and teaching hospitals and departments of pharmacy, and has established relationships and interactions with the Nigerian Association of Industrial Pharmacists (NAIP). The Agency is also working towards integrating Nigerian indigenous natural medicine into the National Healthcare and Management System.

The West African Postgraduate College of Pharmacists (WAPCP)

The West African Postgraduate College of Pharmacists (WAPCP) promotes unstructured interactions between researchers and industry. The Fellows of the College (from both industry and academics) interact with one another during conferences and the annual general meetings of the College, especially during the scientific sessions.

The Nigerian Institute of Medical Research (NIMR)

The Nigerian Institute of Medical Research (NIMR) hardly had any industrial firms relating to it, though the institute expects such interaction to be a two-way affair. If NIMR comes up with an invention that is patented, then the Institute would be in the position to approach firms for its commercialization. Furthermore, NIMR expects that pharma firms should relate with NIMR to inform the institute of their drug production challenges, and provide research funds to resolve such challenges in areas of operation of the institute.

The Pharmaceutical Manufacturing Group of the Manufacturing Association of Nigerian (PMG-MAN)

The Pharmaceutical Manufacturing Group of the Manufacturing Association of Nigerian (PMG-MAN) is the umbrella association of all pharmaceutical manufacturing companies in Nigeria. The Association notes that most Nigerian institutions are not equipped to fill the research gaps in Nigerian Pharmaceutical industry, hence Nigerian companies go to South-East (SE) Asia to consult experts who could solve their problems. A reason that was adduced for this lapse is the content of the syllabus of pharmaceutical studies in Nigerian universities, which was claimed as being inadequate to serve the needs of industry. However, the firms' collaborations with SE Asian countries could possibly have a negative influence on the development of the Nigerian pharmaceutical industry: it is not helpful for the development of a local Pharmaceutical Sector Ecosystem when about 70% of medicines used in Nigeria are imported. One of the goals of PMG-MAN is to reverse the present position of 70% importation against 30% local manufacturing, and increase local production to at least 70%. In addition, to address the deficiency in Nigerian universities, a new curriculum was developed for pharmaceutical studies in line with the needs of industry. This was during a symposium organized in Nigeria by the US Pharmacopeia, and the new curriculum has been launched by the Pharmaceutical Society of Nigeria.

The PMG-MAN on behalf of its members relates with the Nigerian government and other organisations. The PMG-MAN is a member of the West Africa Pharmaceutical Manufacturing Association (WAPMA), which in turn is a member of the Federation of African Pharmaceutical Manufacturing (FAPMAM). FAPMAM contributes to the activities of WHO and the International Association of Pharmaceutical Manufacturers. The Federation holds regional meetings where policies (global, regional and national) that affect member states and challenges confronting them are discussed.

Patents

Besides direct interaction between industrial firms and research organisations, patenting is another avenue through which they can interact. A patent is the protection that is placed on an invention, which confers on the inventor exclusive rights to the industrial exploitation of the invention. Patented inventions enjoy protection from un-authorised commercial exploitation; therefore, the invention cannot be commercially made, used, distributed or sold without the patent owner's consent. Once granted, patent protection generally lasts for 20 years, unless the patent owner does not pay an annual renewal fee; a situation that could result in revocation of the protection. However, with continuous renewal, the protection continues until the expiration of protection time, when such invention enters the public domain and the invention becomes available for free commercial exploitation to the general public.

However, because of the peculiarity of pharmaceutical inventions, their introduction to the market is usually delayed for clinical trials, which delay their entry into the market immediately after they are developed. Therefore, to compensate for the loss of effective patent term caused by regulatory delays in bringing new medicinal products to market, patents for pharmaceutical products may be extended for up to five years by the use of a Supplementary Protection Certificate (SPC). The Drug Price Competition and Patent Term Restoration Act of 1984, usually referred to as the Hatch-Waxman Act, brought about the issuing of SPCs in the USA (Thomas

Database, 2010), while the European Union, Regulation No 1768/92 of 18 June 1992, provides the same for its member countries (EEC, 1992).

Nigerian researchers have not been active in patenting of inventions. WIPO (2017) indicates that in 2016, the total number of patent applications from Nigeria was seven: four through the Patent Cooperation Treaty (PCT) international applications and three through the PCT national phase entry. The total number of applications was too small when compared with figures from other countries, even those from Africa. For instance, applications from Egypt were 2,149; Ghana, 31; Kenya, 203; and South Africa, 9,711. To encourage Nigerian researchers to patent their inventions, the Federal Government of Nigeria, through the National Office for Technology Acquisition and Promotion (NOTAP) in collaboration with the World Intellectual Property Organisation (WIPO), established Intellectual Property Technology Transfer Offices (IPTTOs) in Nigerian tertiary institutions and research institutes. These offices are institutional support structures to assist in the protection and management of intellectual property rights, and to promote interactions and strengthen the linkages between their host institutions and industries. The Offices are also expected to develop robust Intellectual Property Rights (IPR) portfolios through patenting, copyright and technology licensing, and to support the institution's initiative in developing a patent culture. Starting with fifteen that were established in 2006, NOTAP (2020) revealed that 43 IPTTOs have been established in Nigerian universities, polytechnics and research institutes.

Government Policy

Governments worldwide use policies to drive industrial and socio-economic activities in their countries. Such policies are also designed to promote the health and well-being of citizens. In order to promote the development of the pharmaceutical industry in Nigeria, the National Drug Policy (FMoH-WHO, 2005) was launched in 2005. One of the objectives of the policy is to promote pharmaceutical R&D, and develop raw materials for the production, compounding and formulation of pharmaceutical products. The document indicated that drug R&D should be encouraged, especially in the following areas:

i. Local raw materials with particular emphasis on petrochemicals as sources for new drugs and excipients;
ii. Traditional medicines for the promotion of health and the treatment of diseases;
iii. Enhancing the quality and stability of pharmaceutical products;

iv. Documenting and reducing adverse drug reactions.

The policy document did not contain any provision for research on the development of Active Pharmaceutical Ingredients (API), nor on their production. This shows that, as of 2005, the Nigerian government did not see the need to promote the production of API; consequently, industrial firms may find it very difficult to venture into the production of API, when the Government has no plan for its production.

To boost industrial development in the country, the Federal Government of Nigeria drew up the Nigeria Industrial Revolution Plan (FGN, 2014). The plan, which was released on 1 January 2014, was an ambitious national roadmap for industrialisation of the country. This plan intended to create jobs, generate wealth, diversify economy, substitute imports, boost exports, and broaden the tax base, thereby adding about 5 trillion Naira to annual manufacturing revenues in three to five years. The plan focused on developing the sectors where Nigeria has a natural comparative advantage. Unfortunately, the pharmaceutical industry was not included among them. Its omission should not be a shock but should be expected. For instance, Berger et al. (2010) hinted that because pharmaceutical production is capital-intensive and employs relatively few people, it cannot, as an isolated sector, lead to economic development. However, this economic disadvantage of the pharmaceutical industry notwithstanding, efforts should be made to develop the industry because of its strategic importance. Such had been done by some countries in the past. For instance, Dhar et al. (2002) reported that the Indian government used policy to induce the growth of the Indian pharmaceutical industry between the late 1970s and the early 1990s, from its previously relatively small production capacity. Therefore, the FGN should design policies that would strengthen and promote the growth of Nigeria's pharmaceutical industry.

Success Stories of Academic-Industry Linkages in the Pharmaceutical Industry in Nigeria

There are several reports of successful development of inventions from R&D efforts in different fields in Nigeria. In the areas of pharmaceutical R&D, NOTAP (2016) reported the following break-through inventions of raw materials and products:

- Anti-sickling phyto-medicine
- Process for production of pharmaceutical grade starch

- Process for the production of microcrystalline cellulose for use in drug formulation
- Anti-malaria phyto-medicine
- Anti-diabetic phytomedicine
- Anti-fungal phyto-medicine
- Extraction of essential oils from local plants
- Extraction of pharmaceutical grade Artemisinin from Artemisia plants grown in Nigeria

Success Stories of Academic-Industry Technology Transfer in the Pharmaceutical Industry in Nigeria

A major success story of Academic-Industry Technology Transfer in the pharmaceutical industry in Nigeria is Niprisan, a medicine that was developed for the management of sickle cell disease. Niprisan was developed in 1998 by Nigeria's National Institute for Pharmaceutical Research and Development (NIPRD) from medicinal plants that are used for treating the disorder by local traditional herbal medicine producers. The drug passed through clinical studies, was granted a US patent in September 1998, and has been on the market ever since. An "orphan drug" status was secured for Niprisan in the United States in 2004 and in the European Union in 2005.

Before Niprisan was developed, Hydroxyurea was the only approved drug for the treatment of sickle cell, but it was bogged down with multiple concerns about its toxic and carcinogenic side effects on patients. Niprisan is a phytochemical that is formulated from parts of four different indigenous plants namely: *Piper guineenses* (seeds), *Pterocarpus osun* (stem), *Eugenia caryophylum* (fruit) and *Sorghum bicolor* (leaves). Though Niprisan is not a cure for sickle cell anaemia, the drug is useful in managing sickle cell disorder in patents, as it significantly reduces the occurrence of crises without any toxicity or serious adverse effects on patients.

Sickle cell anaemia is a genetic disorder, in which the round red blood cells are deformed so that they become rigid, sticky and are shaped like sickles or crescent moons. Those cells can sometimes lock together, clogging tiny blood vessels or even totally blocking blood flow, thereby preventing some parts of the body from getting oxygen. This situation causes bouts of extreme pain and, sometimes, organ damage to people with the disorder. This occurrence, called sickle cell "crisis", is an intense, unbearable pain all over the body of the patient, and it can last from a few hours to as long as a few weeks, and even result in death. Niprisan reverses the sickling of red blood cells and protects them from becoming sickled when exposed to low oxygen tension. The disease affects over 12 million people of African, Caribbean, or Middle Eastern ancestry, and kills an estimated 50% to 80% of infants born with the disorder before the age of five years.

Unfortunately, the commercialization of Niprisan got hampered by several challenges. The exclusive rights to the patent were sold to a US-based Indian-owned company, Xechem International, in 2003. Xechem established a production plant in Nigeria and the drug was launched into the Nigerian market as Nicosan in 2006. After production slowed down, the exclusive license given to Xechem International for the manufacture and marketing of the drug was withdrawn in March 2009. The Nigerian government took over production through NIPRD but its commercial production was later stopped in 2015. After the patent expired in 2017, an Illinois pharmaceutical company, Xickle started to produce its own version of the drug, which the company claims has twice the anti-sickling activity of the original Niprisan. In order to reactivate the production of the drug in the country, NIPRD signed a production agreement with a Nigerian pharmaceutical company, May & Baker, in June 2018.

Pharmaceutical Technology Transfer in South Africa

Amuasi (2009) reported that South Africa has the most developed pharmaceutical industry in Africa, and is the only African country that produces API and intermediates for the whole of Africa. Several South African pharmaceutical firms had successful technology transfers for pharmaceutical products from foreign technology donors such as Boehringer-Ingelheim, Bristol-Myers Squibb, Gilead Sciences, GlaxoSmithKline, Merck & Co. and Roche AIDS Technology (Berger et al, 2010). Amuasi (2009) further reported that a majority of the over 90 registered pharmaceutical firms operate as sales and marketing offices. Locally produced medicines are mostly generic, and the majority of the production facilities are privately owned. The drivers/incentives identified for Technology Transfer in South Africa include:

- Good business and manufacturing practices
- Potential for competitive pricing
- Strategic planning
- Strong economy, environment and civil society
- Transparent and efficient regulation
- Opportunities for contingency supply
- Public/investor pressure and corporate image

- Access to new machinery, training, know-how and business partnerships

Academia-Industry Linkages in the Indian Pharmaceutical Industry

The transformation of the Indian pharmaceutical industry to its present status took place within a period of about three decades. Dhar et al (2002) suggested that the industry in India evolved through three phases over about 50 years. The first was the period prior to 1970, when the industry was relatively small in terms of production capacities. The second phase spanned the late 1970s to the early 1990s when the industry experienced policy-induced growth, while the third was from the 1990s, when much of the regulatory structure that the government imposed during the previous two decades was dismantled.

The Indian government used decisive policy thrusts to transform the pharmaceutical industry. The policies encouraged the deepening of the production base of the domestic industry by ensuring that the production of drugs took place from the most rudimentary basic stages that are possible. Pharmaceutical firms were also encouraged to embrace R&D by offering various fiscal incentives in the form of tax concessions and exemptions of specific products from the purview of price controls. For instance, the pharmaceutical industry was eligible for a weighted deduction for R&D expenses up to 150%. In addition, the government provided an intellectual property environment that was conducive. In 1970, India adopted a new Patents Act, which became effective from 1972. The new Patents Act replaced the Patents and Designs Act of 1911. Three provisions in Act that benefited the pharmaceutical industry were:

(i) patents could be taken only for processes and not for products;
(ii) patent term of five years from its being granted or seven years from application, whichever was shorter;
(iii) possible issuance of automatic licenses of right three years after the granting of the patent.

The most important of these provisions is the process patent regime that encouraged reverse engineering and the development of alternative processes for the products patented in other countries. Consequently, the firms succeeded in gaining practical experience under the protection of law and were able to acquire production capabilities based on indigenously generated technological activities. This is the principal reason for the growth of the Indian pharmaceutical industry during the 1990s. To enable them to move up the ladder of quality production, Indian firms started paying attention to good manufacturing practices, and their production facilities obtained the approval of the Food and Drug Administration (FDA) of the United States and the Medicines Control Agency (MCA) of the United Kingdom (ICRA, 1999).

A key aspect of technological change in the pharmaceutical sector in India is the close interaction between the industrial firms and the three publicly funded laboratories of the Council for Scientific and Industrial Research (CSIR): the National Chemical Laboratory (NCL) located in Pune; the Central Drug Research Institute (CDRI) located in Lucknow; and the Indian Institute of Chemical Technology (IICT) located in Hyderabad. These interactions led to intense networking between academia, government and industry, and they resulted in the funnelling of intellectual and other resources towards significant incremental progress.

As the firms became well established and innovative, the Indian government adopted a product patent regime that is consistent with the WTO TRIPS Agreement on pharmaceuticals in 2005. The TRIPS agreement was not only for processes but also for products, and the term of protection available is 20 years from the date of filing. Furthermore, the TRIPS Agreement established detailed conditions for compulsory licensing or government use of patents without the authorization of the patent owner.

Lessons from the experience of South Africa and India

To enable Nigeria and other developing countries to develop their pharmaceutical industries, they could learn some lessons from the experiences of South Africa and India. The two countries used different strategies to attain the states their pharmaceutical industries have achieved. South African firms entered into strategic partnerships with well-established foreign pharmaceutical companies, which empowered them to make successful technology transfers. The development is mainly private-sector-driven, as most of the South African pharmaceutical companies are privately-owned. In the case of India, government policies were used to drive pharmaceutical R&D through the reverse engineering of patented medicines, which were developed through alternative processes in government research institutes in collaboration with industrial firms. These practices enabled the firms to gain practical experiences in R&D for the development of medicines.

These show that industrial development could be achieved through diverse means. While the government designs fiscal and non-fiscal policies that would encourage industrial involvement in R&D, industrial firms should be ready to invest in in-house R&D and contract R&D with knowledge institutions such as research institutes and universities. There is also the need for collaboration between firms and institutions to enable them to relate effectively. Consequently, with adequate interactions between industrial firms and knowledge institutions, it is possible for developing countries to achieve the development of their pharmaceutical industries.

CHAPTER SIX

HUMAN RESOURCE DEVELOPMENT FOR THE PHARMACEUTICAL MANUFACTURING SECTOR

ELIZABETH A. OMIMAKINDE

Introduction

Sufficient numbers of highly trained and seasoned professionals are indispensable for a robust national health system in the twenty-first century (Mosadeghrad, 2014). This underscores the need for the assessment of human resource status in Nigeria's pharmaceutical manufacturing sector.

A. Current Human Resource Situation in the Nigerian Pharmaceutical Industry

Registered and Licensed Pharmacists and Pharmacy Technicians in Nigeria

Recent data from the Pharmacists Council of Nigeria indicated an upsurge in the number of registered and licensed pharmacists in the country as their number increased from 20,507 in 2015 to 24,830 in 2018 (Table 6.1). Likewise, the number of annual licences to practice increased from 11,837 in 2015 to 13,304 in 2018. Similarly, there were consistent increases in the number of registered pharmacy technicians and persons who had permits to operate between 2015 and 2018.

This observation is consistent with what was reported by Ekpenyong et al., 2018. They confirmed a rise in the number of pharmacists and new pharmacy graduates per year per 10,000 population over the five years (2011-2016) that were analysed. The increase could be attributed to an increase in the number of pharmacy training institutions in the country.

Table 6.1: Statistics of Registered and Licensed Pharmacists and Pharmacy Technicians in Nigeria

Year	2015	2016	2017	2018
Registered Pharmacists	20, 507	21, 892	23, 437	24, 830
Licensed Pharmacists	11, 837	13, 020	13, 457	13, 304
Registered Pharmacy Technicians	2, 653	3, 131	4, 179	5, 793
Technicians with Annual Permit	249	676	992	2, 204

Source: PCN, 2019

A breakdown of the 2018 statistics (Table 6.2) revealed the gender and geopolitical distributions of licensed Nigerian pharmacists. The geopolitical distribution shows that the majority of the pharmacists are from the South-West (5,507), while the South-East has the least number (1,276). Also from the table, 115 pharmacists who were trained abroad were inducted and licensed to practice in Nigeria after successful completion of the Foreign Graduate Orientation Programme and necessary examinations. The table further shows that a total of 7,770 male and 5,534 female pharmacists were licensed in the same year.

Table 6.2: Distribution of Licensed Pharmacists in Nigeria by Geopolitical zones and Gender

Geopolitical Zone	Geopolitical Zone		Total
	Male	Female	
North-Central	1,785	1,113	2,898
North-East	389	127	516
North-West	662	257	919
South-East	776	500	1,276
South-South	1,096	977	2,073
South-West	2,996	2,511	5,507
Abroad	66	49	115
Total	7,770	5,534	13,303

Source: Data obtained from the PCN during the field survey. This data is for a period of January to December, 2018.

Most of the licensed pharmacists with a known area of practice in Nigeria are in community and hospital practice, with a limited number in academia, industry and administrative pharmacy. This shows that there is a significant deficit in the three latter areas of pharmacy practice in the country. Efforts should be made to address the human resource deficits in these areas.

More has to be done to absorb the available pharmaceutical professionals into the workforce, particularly in the subdivisions where there are significant deficits such as industrial and academic pharmacies. Despite the fact that the number of graduates produced in Nigeria is on the increase, the overall density of pharmacists per 10,000 population remains significantly low, indicating a continuing deficit in pharmaceutical manpower compared to developed countries. For instance, Ekpenyong et al. (2018) reported that the number of Nigeria's pharmacists per 10,000 population in 2016 was approximately 0.7 compared with South Africa (2.7), and the UK (8.08). However, it is hoped that, with the establishment of more pharmacy schools in the country, there will be an increase in the number of qualified and registered pharmacists to fill this gap (Ogaji and Ojabo, 2014; Drame et al., 2019).

From the field survey, 28 pharmaceutical firms responded to the question addressing availability of personnels. Nine (32%) of the firms reported a shortage of staff, seven (25%) reported they have a sufficient number, 12 (43%) firms were not sure. Although only nine firms affirmed a shortage of personnels, 16 firms thereafter gave reasons for their staff shortages. Five (31%) of them reported non-availability of qualified personnels as the cause of their staff shortage, while the remaining 11 (69%) attributed the challenge to insufficient funds.

Though only 31% of the firms reported non-availability of qualified personnel as the reason for their staff shortage, information from a key informant unveiled a shortage in the supply of highly trained production pharmacists is one of the major problems confronting pharma firms in Nigeria. The key informant also disclosed that Nigeria might not be able to boast of more than 200 production pharmacists, for a population of over 200 million. The informant went further and revealed that whenever a fresh pharmacy graduate is employed as a production pharmacist, such personnel still need to undergo training in industry for one or two years, because the training received in pharmacy schools is not very relevant to industrial production.

Another great challenge facing the availability of skilled personnel in the Nigerian pharmaceutical industry is the problem of a brain drain, leading to the exodus of skilled health personnel out of the country. Many Nigerian pharmacists who travel abroad for postgraduate studies end up being employed in their host countries. A study on the financial implications of health personnel emigrating from sub-Saharan Africa revealed that a large number of health personnel from sub-Saharan African countries are employed in the United Kingdom, Australia, Canada and the United States. The actual numbers are estimated by various parties to be in their thousands, and they account for an estimated loss of return on investment of almost US $2.17 billion for West African countries, while the net gain for the developed countries to which they emigrated was estimated to be about US $4.55 billion (UNIDO, 2012).

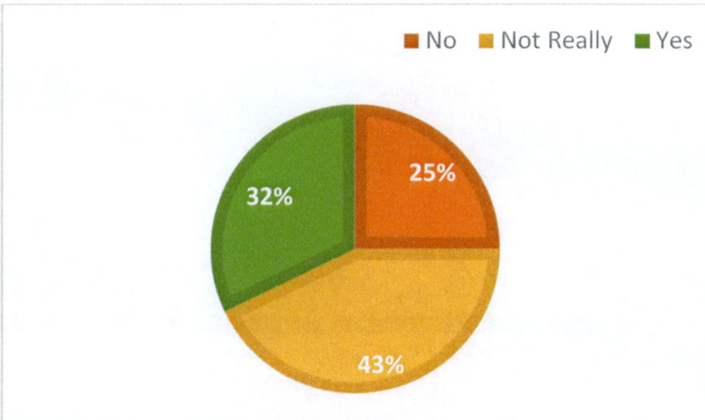

Figure 6.1: Shortage of Personnel in Nigerian Pharma Firms

In order to address the problem of staff shortage, pharma firms either engage the service of part-time workers (50%) or contract staff (50%). Some organizations such as the African Capacity Building Initiative and Carnegie African Diaspora Fellowship program are trying to address this problem of a brain drain and harness the capacity of Africans (including Nigerians) in the diaspora. This is by guiding and building the research expertise and capacity training of this African diaspora towards the continent (Hofman and Kramer, 2015; Langa, 2018). In addition, PCN is also expediting actions on the accreditation of faculties and departments, including specialized institutions providing pharmacy-related courses in the country. For instance, the foreign graduate orientation programme is now being run twice in a year (September and March of every year) to accommodate pharmacists who graduate from various foreign universities. Moreover, during our visit to the Council (PCN), we witnessed the induction of about 150 pharmacists who were trained abroad. Additionally, more universities have approached the PCN for accreditation of their Faculties of Pharmacy.

Nationalities and Professional Affiliation of Staff Members

The nationalities of personnel of Nigerian pharma firms who responded to the study are presented in Figure 6.2. The result reveals that over 97% of the personnel are Nigerians, while the remaining (less than 3%) are from other African, Asian and European countries. The employment of foreigners by the firms shows that they possessed the required skill by the industries. 52% of the surveyed firms reported staff members from Europe and Asia nationalities.

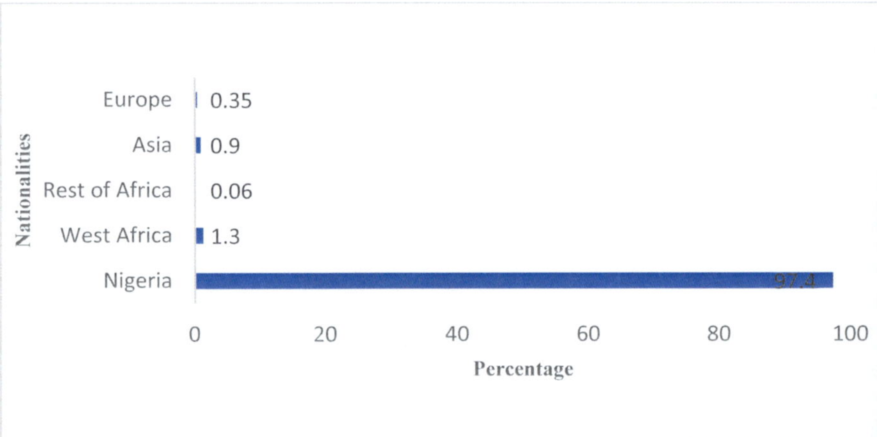

Figure 6.2: Nationalities of Personnel in Nigerian Pharma Firms
Source: Field Study

The employment of personnel of foreign nationalities could indicate reliance of the firms on the expertise of foreign technology suppliers. Though above 90% of the personnel are Nigerians, their highest educational qualifications presented in Figure 6.3 revealed most of them may not play core technical roles in the companies.

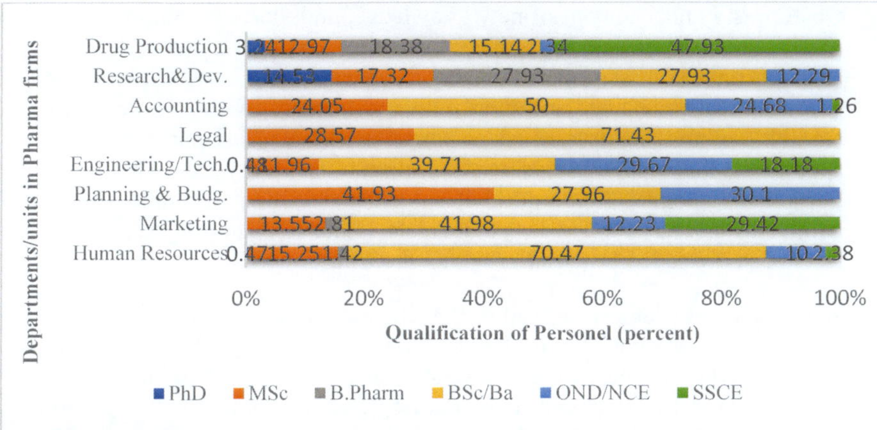

Figure 6.3: Highest Qualifications of Personnel in Nigeria Pharma Firms
Source: Field survey

Highest Qualifications of Staff in Nigerian Pharmaceutical firms

Regarding the educational attainment and training obtained by the workers, a large number of personnel in the pharma firms have bachelor's degrees. Some others have master's, while only a few in Research and Development (R&D) and Drug Production Departments have doctorate degrees (Figure 6.3). This result is a pointer to the level of capabilities available in the industry. The educational capability of available R&D staff equally points to the level of research activities in industrial firms. For instance, research-based postgraduate education has been observed to play a key role in the propensity to innovate and develop more robust capacities in R&D activities, as a result of the scientific research experience acquired in the course of the programme (Lam, 2005; Wang et al., 2019). This implies that better R&D outputs would be obtained where R&D staff have master's or doctoral degrees (Wendler et al., 2010; Cele and Lekhnaya, 2016). Among Nigerian pharma firms that responded to this study, first university degrees were the most prominent highest academic qualifications amongst the staff. The breakdown according to departments is hereafter discussed briefly.

Research and Development Department: The need for R&D in the pharmaceutical industry cannot be overemphasized. A great deal of R&D is conducted to develop new medicines and improve existing ones by pharmacists and scientists all over the world. R&D activities demand a huge investment in technical and human capital resources, culminating in the creation and enhancement of new knowledge, and thereby leading to new or improved products and processes. The pharmaceutical industry depends on R&D in all its stages, from drug discovery to the development and production of medicines and their delivery processes. None of these are possible without highly trained personnel in the R&D department, with appropriate knowledge. As presented in Figure 6.3, among the 16 pharma firms that responded to the question on personnel, the percentage of PhD holders in those firms was less than 15 % (14.53%). This suggests a low level of in-house R&D activities within the firms.

Nevertheless, as later discussed in this chapter, Nigerian universities have been training students for bachelor's, master's and doctorate degrees in Pharmaceutical Studies over the years. However, several of the trained pharmacists have emigrated in search of better wages and conditions of service outside Nigeria. Consequently, Ekeigwe (2019) reported that there is a scarcity of indigenous skilled technical personnel for drug development and production in Nigeria. This paucity of trained and competent personnel is affecting all areas of the pharmaceutical ecosystem: the academic, regulatory, and manufacturing fields.

Marketing Department: A large proportion (44.79%) of the personnel in this department among respondents were first-degree holders, who had acquired degrees in various disciplines. It is noteworthy that this department engaged the service of the largest number of MSc and BSc/BA holders; and the third largest percentage of B. Pharm holders in the pharma industry. These personnel serve as sales representatives of the pharma firms. Pharmaceutical sales representatives secure transactions for their company's pharmaceutical products. Their business is to convince medical professionals that the medications, treatments and expedients that they offer are perfect for their patient's needs and superior to those offered by their competitors. Pharmaceutical companies frequently send their representatives to meet with doctors to offer free product samples, deliver information about product use and to answer the doctors' questions (McNeill, 2006). The employment of B. Pharm holders in their marketing departments shows that the firms engage professional pharmacists to present their products to the market to enable them to capture market niche.

Human Resource Management (HRM) Department: The HRM department works in support of the development and growth of the company through the recruitment of suitable personnel for the company, and by getting the best applicants to make the company grow faster (Biotechnology Community, 2018). A good percentage (87%) of personnel in this department had university degrees (Figure 6.3). This result suggests that the HRM department has one of the strongest teams of personnel in the industry. This strength would enable the department to perform its duties of recruiting and retaining the best employees.

Engineering/Technical Department (ETD): These departments are responsible for designing, building, operating, innovating and improving manufacturing facilities for the production of a company's products. More specifically, a standard ETD must be able to handle the increasingly complex requirements of Good Manufacturing Practice (GMP) to ensure the safety of the drugs their companies produce. The field survey revealed that about 52% of the personnel in this department possessed a minimum of BSc/BEng certificates, 29% were OND/NCE holders, while 18% were holders of SSCE (Figure 6.3). The engineers, who constitute over half of the personnel, were the backbone of the technical department, while others serve as technical assistants and attendants supporting the engineers in their activities.

Account and Finance (A&F) Department: The Account and Finance (A&F) department is one of the major pillars of a vibrant pharmaceutical organisation and an essential ingredient to a successful business. The A&F department has a broad range of roles to carry out within and outside the organization. Pharma firms, being capital-intensive organizations, their performance and success greatly depend on how well their finance is handled. Therefore, a robust A&F department is very essential for the smooth running of pharma firms.

24% of the personnel in the A&F department of Nigeria's pharma firms were MSc holders, 50% were BSc/BA holders, and 25% were non-degree holders. These data suggest that the A&F departments of Nigerian pharma firms are manned by well-qualified personnel.

***Planning and Budgeting Department*:** This department is responsible for making financial plans to help managers direct and manage companies' operations and activities (Kovaleva et al., 2016). The highest number of the staff in this department has a master's degree (41; 93%); 27.96% and 30% possessed a first degree and either an NCE or OND certificate, respectively (Figure 6.3 above).

***Legal Unit*:** The Legal Units of pharmaceutical firms handle matters on the protection, acquisition and management of intellectual properties (IPs) such as patents and trademarks. The unit also works on a firm's licensing and takes legal action over any infractions of the rights the firms may have over the IPs. As presented in Figure 6.3, 29% of the personnel in this unit of surveyed pharma firms were Masters of Law (LLM) holders, while the rest were Bachelors of Law (LLB) holders. However, out of the 32 sampled firms, only 11 responded to this question. This suggests that most of the firms might not have an in-house legal department, but outsource to law firms to handle their legal matters.

Professional Affiliations of the Workforce: 30 firms answered the question on certification of personnel by the Pharmaceutical Council of Nigeria (PCN) and other professional bodies in Nigeria, including the Council for the Regulation of Engineering in Nigeria (COREN). The responses of the firms are presented in Figure 6.4. Certification of staff by PCN had the highest percentage (62.45%) and this is expected because pharmacists are the core staff of pharmaceutical firms and they cannot operate without the certification. Affiliation with other professional bodies like the Institute of Chartered Accountants of Nigeria (ICAN), the Nigerian Society of Engineers (NSE), the Nigeria Institute of Management (NIM) etc. were subsumed under the bodies indicated as "Others", though the research instrument was not specific about them.

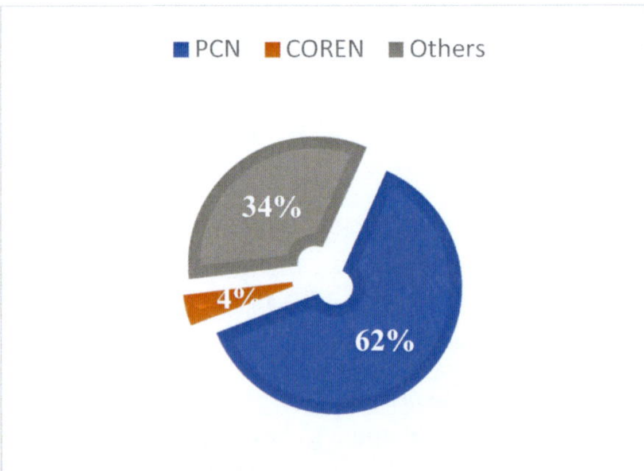

Figure 6.4: Professional Affiliation of Nigerian Pharma Workforce
Source: Field survey

B. Training of Pharmacists in Nigeria

i. Universities

The pharmaceutical industry, known for its high R&D intensity, requires highly trained workforce. Hence, Stephane et al. (2006) emphasised sufficient numbers of highly trained and seasoned professionals are essential for a robust health system. To provide these services, the Nigerian government has been making a huge investment in the training of pharmacists at different levels.

Nigeria has a total of 75 Federal and State-owned universities located across all the thirty-six states and the Federal Capital Territory, Abuja. Out of these institutions, 23 are offering programmes in pharmaceutical fields, and 20 of them were already accredited by the Pharmacists Council of Nigeria (PCN) as of year 2021 (PCN, 2021). These universities function mainly to train students for bachelor's, master's and doctorate degrees in pharmaceutical programmes, to provide the much-needed human resource for the pharmaceutical sub-sector. In the four years studied, from 2015 to 2018, these universities produced over 12,000 pharmacists, including those practising locally and outside the country. The numbers of graduates from the institutions in each of these years are presented in Figure 6.5.

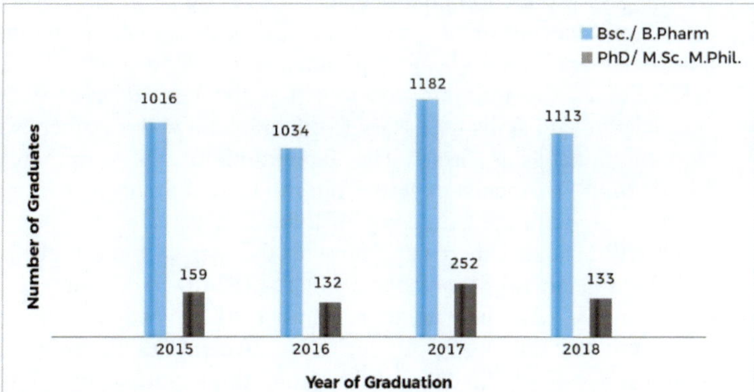

Figure 6.5: Number of Pharmacists Trained in Nigeria between 2015 and 2018
Source: Field Survey, 2019

ii. Other Training Organizations in Nigeria

In addition to faculties of pharmacy in Nigerian universities, professional pharmaceutical associations also play key roles in the training and re-training of pharmacists. The roles of these organisations are briefly discussed below:

1. **Pharmacists Council of Nigeria (PCN):** The training, registration and licensing of pharmacists in Nigeria are regulated by the PCN, as well as accreditation of pharmacy training schools. (As stated above, 23 universities offer pharmaceutical studies, and 20 have been accredited by the PCN). However, the universities that have not been accredited for the course have approached the PCN for their accreditation and the process is on-going. PCN is also expediting actions on the accreditation of faculties and departments, including specialized institutions providing pharmacy-related courses in the country. For instance, the foreign graduate orientation programme is being run twice a year to accommodate those pharmacists who have graduated from various foreign universities. The first batch comes during the first quarter of each year and the subsequent group comes up during the last quarter of every year.
2. **Association of Industrial Pharmacists in Nigeria (NAIP)**: The Association of Industrial Pharmacists in Nigeria (formerly known as the Nigerian Association of Industrial Pharmacists) is involved in the training of production pharmacists. The Association has in the past sponsored seven of its members for postgraduate programmes (master's and postgraduate diplomas) at the University of Ibadan. The aim of the training was to equip the beneficiaries with the knowledge and skills necessary to enable them to train others within the manufacturing firms. The facilitators of the program were production pharmacist experts from the United States of America in partnership with the University of Ibadan, Nigeria.

   NAIP academy also came up with the idea of the establishment of Pharmaceutical Manufacturing Parks (PMP) in different parts of the country, and has made a number of advocacies with state governments including Ogun, Oyo, Anambra, Ebonyi, Kano. Interestingly, as at the time of compiling this report, a key informant from the association mentioned during the interview that two states of the Federation have made lands available and also promised to provide the projects with some infrastructure. One of the objectives of the park is massive production of pharmaceutical products for export, to enable Nigeria to participate maximally in the continental trade agreement coming up soon in the country. NAIP has also planned to undertake massive training of production pharmacists who would work in these PMP.

3. **Nigeria Association of Pharmacists and Pharmaceutical Scientists in the Americas (NAPPSA):** The Pharmaceutical Society of Nigeria (PSN) confirmed the Society is working with NAPPSA. This collaboration has resulted in the commencement of a Special Doctor of Pharmacy (Pharm D.) programme at the University of Benin, Edo State, Nigeria. One key informant also mentioned the involvement of members of NAPPSA in this training and the upgrading of the knowledge of practising B. Pharm holders to Pharm D. The PSN is also organising a fellowship programme, whereby NAPPSA members would make working visits to Nigeria, help to build local capacity and transfer knowledge both to pharmacists in the industry and to those in academia.
4. **Association of Community Pharmacists of Nigeria (ACPN):** Community Pharmacists have direct involvement in the training of young pharmacists. ACPN members work in collaboration with the PCN in conducting accreditation exercises in universities to regulate pharmacy education in Nigeria. ACPN members are also involved in teaching (lecturing) in the faculties of pharmacy of some universities. For instance, some ACPN members were regularly involved in the teaching of practical pharmaceutical practices at the University of Port Harcourt. ACPN members are also participating in the training of graduate pharmacists, who undergo a compulsory one-year internship training programme after their five years of regular university study before going for the National Youth Service Corps programme. Some community pharmacy centres have been approved by PCN for this purpose. It was gathered during the interview that some ACPN members had some interns under their close supervision, while a pharma firm was reported to have over 30 interns undergoing training within the establishment.
5. ***Contributions of Nigerian Pharmacists in the Diaspora to the Development of the Nigerian Pharmaceutical Sector:*** The survey also examined the contributions of the Nigerian Pharmacists in the Diaspora (NPD) to the development of the Nigerian pharmaceutical sub-sector. 69 university pharmacy researchers responded to this question. 50 (72.5%) respondents declared there were no contributions from NPD whatsoever, but seven (10%) affirmed their efforts, while five (7%) were not sure of any support from them. These responses indicate that the support of Nigerian Pharmacists in the Diaspora has

not been felt by many of the researchers in the field of pharmacy in Nigeria. The respondents who received support from NPD indicated book donation, donation of facilities to institutions, funding of research projects, the teaching of undergraduate and postgraduate students and sponsorship to conferences as the areas where they have enjoyed such support.

C. Success Story of the Indian Pharmaceutical Industry and Some Pertinent Lessons for the Development of the Nigerian Pharmaceutical Industry

India's pharmaceutical industry was valued at $41 billion in 2021 and is estimated to increase to $65 billion by 2024 (Economic Survey, 2020-21). The success of the Indian pharmaceutical industry is hailed all over the world. Regarded as a highly competitive and cut-throat sector, the Indian pharma companies have been able to survive competition with big firms in Europe and America in many ways. As of 2021, more than 500,000 people were employed in India's pharma sector (Perlitz et al., 2008) in over 12,000 firms, out of which over 3,000 are big companies. Though drug prices in India are much cheaper than in Europe and the US, these companies are still thriving. Some of the secrets of the competitive edge of Indian companies include:

***Production of Cost-effective Generic Drugs*:** Indian pharmaceutical firms succeeded in the production of generic drugs through reverse engineering and development of brand-name products, through alternative processes by highly trained manpower. The drugs are usually produced at much lower costs thereby making their prices lower and more affordable. India became the third-largest drug manufacturer in the world due to its ability to manufacture highly efficient generic drugs (Akhtar, 2013). India's track record of low-cost development of chemical synthesis for various drug molecules is excellent, and the country has succeeded in producing a wide variety of bulk drugs for local consumption and export.

***Export to the West*:** One of the major reasons for the sustainability and performance of the Indian pharma industry is exporting to the Western world. The availability of cheap generic drugs led many suppliers from the West to outsource production from Indian pharmaceutical firms, and the small and medium-sized Indian firms were able to meet the demands. It is remarkable to note that the US is the largest market for Indian pharma companies.

***Government Support*:** Indian pharmaceutical companies enjoyed strong backing from the government and this has encouraged the industry to excel. Beginning with a patent regime that encouraged the development and production of generic drugs, the Indian government investment environment encouraged the inflow of foreign direct investment, and the pharma industry was able to absorb over 70% of the investments. The good business environment made it easy for Indian businesses to draw in investors and invest more in the industry (Joshi, 20003).

***Backup from the IT sector*:** India's IT sector specializes in providing exceptional service at affordable rates. Having already given people and organisations in the Western world confidence in their performance, the Indian IT industry became the trailblazer that cleared the path for pharmaceutical companies. Consequently, European and American companies did not hesitate to have confidence in partnering with the Indian pharma industry, based on the trust they already had with the Indian IT companies.

***Globalization*:** Globalization also helped Indian pharma firms to attract business contract offers from the USA and Europe. As business organisations seek cheaper products and services, they look beyond the borders of their countries and contract their operations to offshore companies that can provide them with the products and services they produce or provide, at the right quality. This situation gave Indian pharma firms the opportunities to produce for international supply, pressure which enabled the firms to scale up from small firms to medium-sized and then large-sized firms.

In summary, the Indian government provides a conducive environment for pharma companies to produce at low cost, and also encourages the inflow of foreign direct investment into the country.

D. The Extent to which Nigeria with a Relatively More Developed Pharmaceutical Sector Can Help Other West African Countries to Develop Their Local Pharmaceutical Industries

Nigeria produces about 60% of the volume of pharmaceutical products consumed in the Economic Community of West African States (ECOWAS), a community with an estimated population of about 600 million (WHO, 2014). Even with this level of exports, the capacity utilization of Nigerian pharma firms is about 40% (UNIDO, 2011). With increased demand from the ECOWAS countries, the large volume of under-utilized manufacturing capacity could be applied in more production, which could reduce the average cost of production, and it could also be used for the production of new products, especially for export markets.

From the field survey, approximately 13% of the surveyed pharma firms reported market coverage of Francophone and Anglophone countries in West Africa (Figure 6.6). Incidentally, half of these firms also made claim to possessing production facilities in other African countries. These firms could be encouraged to expand their production bases in those countries to enable them to capture larger market shares. If the companies could achieve this feat, it would make the countries less dependent on importation from Nigeria. By so doing, the pharmaceutical industry in those countries would develop and grow gradually. However, to achieve this goal, the host countries should provide the necessary enabling environment for the firms to thrive.

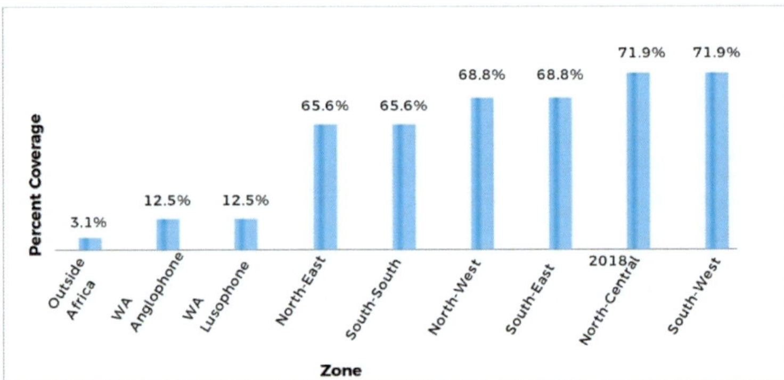

Figure 6.6: Market Coverage of Nigerian Pharma Firms

Source: Field Study

Some characteristics of Nigeria's Pharma Firms

Firm Ownership

Nigerian pharmaceutical firms are mostly indigenous, as 87.50% of them are exclusively owned by Nigerian citizens, 6.3% are jointly owned by foreigners and indigens, and 3.1% are owned by multinational firms (Figure

6.7). These ownership structures are similar to what was earlier reported by Siyanbola et al. (2012), where 60% of the companies were reported to be indigenously owned, 36% belong to foreigners, while 4% were multinationals.

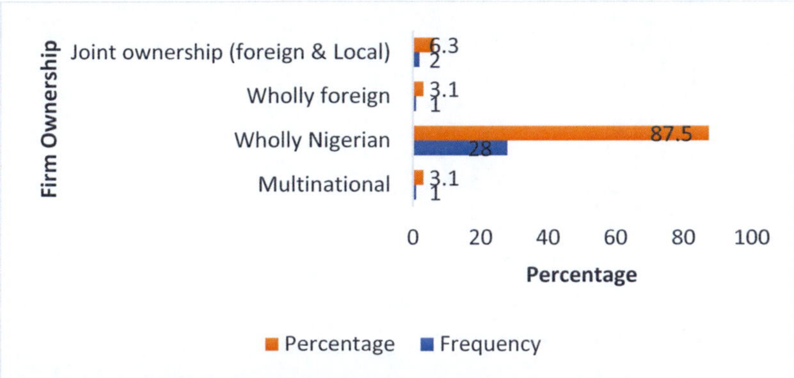

Figure 6.7: Ownership of Nigerian Pharmaceutical Firms Covered in the Study
Source: Field Study

Turnover of the Nigerian Pharmaceutical Firms

Only 22 firms responded to the question addressing their turnover for the year 2018. Figure 6.8 presents the values that were reported by the firms. The figure shows that the company with the least turnover realized four million nairas (₦4 million), while the firm with the highest turnover realized 16 billion naira (₦16 billion). The figure also revealed that the turnovers of two firms were within the range of ₦4 million to ₦10 million, nine firms were within the range of ₦10 million to ₦50 million, one firm was within the range of ₦50 million to ₦100 million, two firms were within the range of ₦100 million to ₦1 billion, six firms were within the range of ₦1 billion to ₦10 billion, while only one firm reported a turnover within the range of ₦10 billion to ₦20 billion. Funding is a critical factor for a robust pharma industry. Many Nigerian pharma firms are small-sized firms that are struggling to survive; consequently, only 30% of them reported an annual turnover of above one billion nairas (₦1,000,000,000).

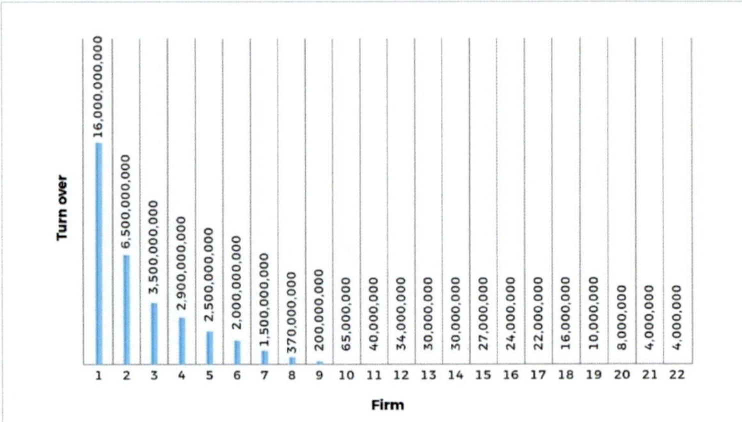

Figure 6.8: Turnover of Nigeria Pharmaceutical Firms in 2018

Source: Field Study

CHAPTER SEVEN

CONCLUSION AND RECOMMENDATIONS

The Nigerian Pharmaceutical Sector- An Overview

The Nigerian pharmaceutical sector is made up of over 200 registered firms, out of which about 120 are involved in the manufacturing of medicinal products. The majority of these firms are small- and medium-sized enterprises, and most of them are owned by Nigerians. Among the respondents, the turnover of the firms for the year 2018 ranged from four million naira (₦4 million) to 16 billion naira (₦16 billion). Most of the staff of Nigerian pharma firms are Nigerians, with a few of them from other West-African countries, Asia and Europe.

It is well-known that huge financial and technological investments are required for the establishment and growth of a sustainable pharma sector, especially where firms have to develop the Active Pharmaceutical Ingredients (API) that are used to produce medicines from the very basic raw materials. However, the Nigerian pharmaceutical sector depends largely on importation of key production inputs, the API and the manufacturing plants. The relatively small size of Nigerian pharmaceutical firms prevents the majority of them from investing in either R&D or the production of API. Consequently, the majority of the firms are not into the real act of drug production: they import API, which they mix, formulate and package as medicines. This challenge notwithstanding, some firms are involved in the production of API for malaria drugs and antacid medication, while two of the firms produce antiretrovirals.

Experience from countries such as India reveals that foreign direct investments (FDIs) are crucial for the development of the pharmaceutical industry, and Nigeria has been having an inflow of investment. For instance, Statista (2022) disclosed that the FDI into Nigeria rose from US $6.03 billion in 2010 to US $8.84 billion in 2011, and gradually declined to US $3.06 billion in 2015. Thereafter, it rose to US $3.45 billion in 2016 and gradually declined to US $0.78 billion in 2018. The figures for 2019 and 2020 were US $2.31 billion and US $2.39 billion respectively. The fall in the inflow of FDI could be a response to the business and economic environment and the general insecurity that prevails in the country. The Nigerian government should therefore address these issues and put in place policy measures that would encourage the inflow of FDIs in order for the pharmaceutical industry to flourish.

An example of a pragmatic policy that could promote the local production of medicines in Nigeria is the "5+5 Policy" that was initiated by the National Agency for Food and Drug Administration and Control (NAFDAC). The policy required that importers of medicines that Nigerian pharma companies have the capacity to produce to commence local production of such drugs after some years of importation. Any company that imports such medicines for five years is mandated to provide a blueprint of how the company would manufacture the same in Nigeria within the next five years. Failure to provide such blueprint within five years of importation could result in sanctions from NAFDAC, as both the company and its imported product would be deregistered or barred from the Nigerian market. This policy made some Indian companies engage Nigerian pharma manufacturing companies in contract manufacturing, while some others are considering establishing subsidiaries in Nigeria. The "5+5 Policy" was initiated when Prof. Dora Akunyili was the Director-General/Chief Executive Officer (DG/CEO) of NAFDAC; it was put on hold by her successor, and later given a push by the next.

The majority of Nigerian pharma firms are yet to acquire WHO prequalification due to the high standards required and the huge financial commitment involved. In May 2023, a pharma firm in Nigeria, with affiliation to a French multinational pharmaceutical company, successfully received WHO prequalification of Zinc Dispersible 20mg Tablet. This is the first company in Africa to obtain WHO prequalification for that medicine. This is a laudable achievement, and further strengthens the fact that with a favorable business infrastructures and policy, the industry has what it takes to compete in the global landscape.

The major impediments to the production of API in the country are not necessarily a lack of human resources and capability, but the huge capital outlay required, and more importantly the absence of a functional petrochemical industry that would provide the necessary raw materials.

The surveyed firms employed pharmacists with qualifications of up to doctorate level. The total number of Pharmacy Council of Nigeria (PCN)-certified pharmacists that were employed by the 32 firms that participated in the survey was 346. The majority of the PhD holders employed in the pharma firms were practising in the R&D departments, while drug production departments reported the highest population of B. Pharm holders. One quarter of the firms surveyed affirmed they have an adequate number of staff, while those without an adequate number of suitably qualified staff attributed this lack to insufficient funds at their disposal; and therefore, resorted to employment of contract and part-time workers.

Between 2014 and 2018, Nigerian universities produced a total of about 8,000 graduate pharmacists and around 800 Master's and Doctorate degrees holders in Pharmaceutical Studies. It was also reported from the survey that a special program to facilitate the training of Pharm D. graduates was organized in the University of Benin through the intervention of the Nigerian Association of Pharmacists and Pharmaceutical Sciences of America (NAPPSA).

The Nigerian Association of Industrial Pharmacists (NAIP) is also working towards resolving the challenge of the dearth of production pharmacists in Nigerian pharma firms, through the provision of scholarships and the training of pharmacists in industrial/production pharmacy. Resource persons for the programme include expert production pharmacists from the United States of America.

The Association of Community Pharmacists of Nigeria (ACPN) in collaboration with PCN usually form part of accreditation panels for pharmacy schools in Nigeria universities. In addition, ACPN members teach in some universities and supervise graduates during their one-year internship programme.

The National Agency for Food and Drug Administration and Control (NAFDAC), the Standards Organisation of Nigeria (SON) and the Pharmacists Council of Nigeria (PCN) play important regulatory roles in the production of quality medicines and other health-care products in Nigeria. NAFDAC regulates and controls food and drugs administration and ensures they meet specified safety levels, SON ensures that the equipment and machinery deployed by the manufacturing companies measure up to the expected standards, while PCN provides guidelines to ensure that competent hands are engaged in pharmaceutical practices and also to ensure that pharma premises meet required standards.

Cost of Medicines

It is well documented that medicines are more expensive in Nigeria than in other African countries, due to a costly supply chain and poor implementation of government policies. Nevertheless, the Bureau for Public Procurement (BPP) Policy of the Government, which is facilitating bulk purchase of medicines and other medicinal products at competitive prices, has reduced the supply chain costs. The policy also stipulates that 70% of essential medicines that are procured by the Nigerian government should be done locally. Besides the BPP, the National Health Insurance Scheme (NHIS) is providing a subsidy that lowers the cost of medicines for its beneficiaries, the majority of whom are public servants. But the policy lacks proper implementation and monitoring, and there is a need for its review to emphasize the procurement of locally manufactured generic medicines. Though the NHIS was expected to achieve national coverage by 2015, only Federal Government employees are currently registered beneficiaries. To complement the NHIS, several states in the country have established similar schemes to cater for their residents.

The "5+5" Policy designed by the National Agency for Food and Drug Administration and Control (NAFDAC) is expected to promote the local production of medicines that are hitherto not produced in Nigeria, but which Nigerian firms have the capability to produce. The production of such medicines is expected to result in their affordability. The small size of most Nigerian pharma firms makes it difficult for them to mobilize the huge resources needed to expand their production and technological capabilities. Consequently, they could not exploit the TRIPS flexibilities to produce some medicines. Furthermore, most of the medicines that are produced by the companies are produced under licenses from foreign multinational pharmaceutical companies. This increases production costs, which also has negative impacts on the price and affordability of medicines in Nigeria.

In summary, the goal of the National Drug Policy, first published in 1990, of making effective, affordable, safe and good quality medicines available to all Nigerians at all times is yet to be realized, decades after its publication.

Research and Development (R&D) Activities

Basic research is the most prominent research activity undertaken by researchers in Nigerian schools of pharmacy, although some conduct drug development research. Lack of funds and infrastructures are the basic bottlenecks hindering drug R&D activities in Nigerian universities.

However, less than half of the Nigerian firms surveyed have functioning in-house R&D departments, and pharmaceutical research accounted for the majority of their R&D activities.

The majority of pharmaceutical researchers in Nigerian universities were not aware of funding organizations that could support their research activities, either at the national, regional or international level. However, a few of the researchers affirmed their awareness; and some of them were granted research funds by international organizations within the last five years. Unlike in the OECD countries where most of the R&D funding is provided by the private sector, less than 10% of the pharmaceutical researchers received funds for research from that sector. This was attributed to obsolete research infrastructure, including laboratories, and inadequate and irregular funding of the institutions, among other reasons.

From the survey, the greatest source of R&D funds used by pharma researchers was personal funds, followed by the government through the Tertiary Education Trust Fund, and university research grants, while grants received from pharma firms were considered to be infinitesimal in nature. This attests to weak interaction between the duo, especially in terms of funding of R&D.

At a regional level, the Africa Research Exchange Funds and the Africa Academy of Science have been involved in the funding of pharmaceutical research activities in Nigeria, while the United Nations International Children's Emergency Fund (UNICEF) and World Bank are involved at a global level. In addition, less than one quarter of pharmaceutical researchers at Nigerian universities have ever received research grants from non-government organisations (NGOs). The chief reason for this was the researchers' inability to explore the available funding opportunities. All the R&D activities conducted by Nigerian pharmaceutical firms were sponsored by the firms individually.

Almost the entire API used by Nigerian pharmaceutical firms to formulate medicines are being imported from China and India, while some were brought in from Germany and the United Kingdom. The few that are produced in-house by the firms were for anti-malaria and antacid medicines. The major impediments hindering the local production of API were identified as lack of political will by the government, paucity of funds, poor infrastructures, absence of a petrochemical raw material base. Other factors are WHO certification and intellectual property issues.

The research activities of Nigerian research institutes in medicine and health-related products have yielded several outcomes. For instance, several research projects by the Raw Materials Research and Development Council, on the development of local materials for use by the pharma firms, were successful. The National Institute for Pharmaceutical Research and Development also reported successful development of several medications. Similarly, the Nigeria Natural Medicine Development Agency recorded successful development of some herbal therapies and nutritional supplements. The agency also developed a mosquito repellent cream, an antimalarial herbal tea, and a supplement for the management of HIV/AIDS. Successful development of these breakthroughs notwithstanding, the inventions have not been taken up by pharma firms for commercial production. It is therefore necessary to put in place some policies to encourage commercialization of these findings. As part of its research efforts, the Nigeria Institute of Medical Research (NIMR) initiated efficacy testing on recommended antimalarial drugs in three states in Nigeria. It also conducted an entomological survey targeting malaria elimination through mosquito eradication. NIMR is also undertaking a programme to design self-testing kits for HIV/AIDS.

The Nigerian government is not ready for the local production of API, as can be deduced from NDP (2005) and the NIRP (2014). Therefore, it is very difficult for firms to venture into its production. However, some breakthroughs were reported by NOTAP in the area of phyto-medicine products. An example of this class of medicine is NIPRISAN, which was the developed in 1998 by NIPRID in collaboration with local herbal medicine practitioners.

Nigeria should learn from the experience of South Africa, where high-level commitment, collaboration and strategic partnerships of local firms with well-established foreign pharmaceutical companies enabled the local South African firms to develop. A key aspect of technological change in the pharmaceutical sector in India is a government policy which stimulated strong interaction between private sector pharmaceutical firms and public research institutes. These interactions led to intense networking between academia, government and industry, and resulted in the development of generic medicines through reverse engineering.

It is also worth mentioning that some pharma firms succeeded in developing some medicines based on Nigerian indigenous knowledge and biodiversity for the treatment of malaria. However, the small size of Nigerian pharma firms makes it impossible for them to mobilize the huge resources needed for pharma R&D. Most of the products sold in the country are under the license of foreign multinational pharmaceutical firms and this among other reasons has resulted in high prices, thereby negatively affecting the affordability of medicines in Nigeria. In addition, the local firms lack the technological capability to exploit the TRIPS flexibilities to produce essential medicines, so the country has to rely on their importation, thereby contributing to the non-affordability of these medicines.

A large number of research outputs from Nigerian universities and research institutes remain unexploited. The route for dissemination of the research outputs of Nigerian pharmaceutical researchers, in order of prevalence, is journal articles, books, and technical reports. None of the respondents reported having patented any research output. To address the poor culture of patenting of inventions among Nigerian researchers, the National Office for Technology Acquisition and Promotion (NOTAP), in collaboration with the World Intellectual Property Organisation (WIPO), has established Intellectual Property Technology Transfer Offices (IPTTOs) in Nigerian universities, polytechnics and research institutes.

Interaction and Collaboration

The level of interaction and collaboration between the firms and knowledge institutions and indigenous herbal medicine producers is low. However, the few firms that collaborated with research institutions enjoyed beneficial collaborations, which were moderately strong. On their part, over 30% of the researchers rated their collaborations with pharmaceutical firms to be at least moderately strong, while close to 70% rated the collaborations to be at least weak. The areas of collaboration include knowledge sharing, provision of R&D services, students' industrial attachment programmes and research consultancy, among others. The majority of the joint R&D activities between firms and research organizations were directed towards malaria and very few are focused on HIV/AIDS. The pharma firms also have collaborations for capacity building and contract manufacturing among themselves.

Other forms of collaborations were revealed by the study. The Nigeria Natural Medicine Development Agency (NNMDA) had established collaborations with the Nigerian Association of Industrial Pharmacists (NAIP), and is collaborating with firms for the commercialization of its research outputs. The Pharmaceutical Society of Nigeria (PSN) in collaboration with the US Pharmacopeia developed a new curriculum for Nigerian pharma schools to address the deficiency in the curriculum that is presently being used, and is also collaborating with the National Association of Pharmacists in Academia (NAPA) and the National Association of Industrial Pharmacist (NAIP) to develop pharmaceutical-grade starch, colorant, and adjuvant excipients and other substrates from local raw materials for use in manufacturing in order to replace imported ones. The Association is also sourcing funds from industry to enable academics to develop API, and a master plan and business feasibility study had been drawn up for the endeavour. The Pharmaceutical Manufacturing Group of Manufacturers Association of Nigeria (PMG-MAN), as the umbrella organization for Nigerian pharmaceutical firms, is the spokesman of Nigerian pharma manufacturers. The association relates with the Government, and with regional, continental and international organisations on behalf of members to assist them in their operations.

Concluding Remarks

Nigeria is the largest producer of pharmaceutical products in West Africa and as well the largest importer of the products. Pharmaceutical imports of the country were estimated to be about US $1.45 billion in 2019.[1] The majority of Nigerian pharmaceutical manufacturing firms are small- and medium-sized enterprises, which lack the financial capacity to engage in the real act of drug production, but mainly mix imported API, and formulate and package the resulting medicines. Therefore, to enable them to scale up, the Nigerian government should intervene with the establishment of a Pharmaceutical Industry Development Fund, which willing pharmaceutical manufacturing firms could access at a low interest rate.

Such a fund would provide an incentive to the firms and enable them to work towards acquiring WHO prequalification for their products. The acquisition of the prequalification would encourage the firms to engage more of their idle capacities. The fund could also be used to support the "5+5" policy of NAFDAC, which would tend to boost local production of medicine in Nigeria, if given the necessary political support by the government. The policy compels the importer of a medicine that Nigerian pharma firms have the capacity to produce to provide a blueprint of how the company intends to manufacture it within five years of its importation, and to commence local production or engage in contract production within another five years.

Nigeria has the potential to establish itself as the leading manufacturer and distributor of essential medicines in sub-Saharan Africa. With its fairly

[1] https://tradingeconomics.com/nigeria/imports/pharmaceutical-products

robust technical skills, averagely trained manpower and basic manufacturing infrastructure already in existence, the country could move up the ladder of industrial development in the pharmaceutical industry. This feat could be achieved with policy interventions, such as those that promote industrial funding of research, interactions between the pharmaceutical firms and researchers in knowledge institutions, and adequate funding of research activities. In addition, increased R&D efforts in the universities and research institutes could lead to the development of new chemical substances, formulations, therapeutic agents, nutraceuticals and phytomedicines from the abundant indigenous biodiversity and traditional medicine in Nigeria.

REFERENCES

Adewole, D.A, Adebayo, A.M, Udeh, E.I., Shaahu, V.N., and Dairo, M.D. "Payment for Health Care and Perception of the National Health Insurance Scheme in a Rural Area in Southwest Nigeria". *Am J Trop Med Hyg.*93, No. 3, (2015):648-54. doi: 10.4269/ajtmh.14- 0245. Epub 2015 Jul 20. PMID: 26195464; PMCID: PMC4559712.

Adewopo, A. "Public health, access to medicines and the role of patents system in Nigeria". NIALS *Journal of Intellectual Property*, Maiden edition (2011):165-190.

Akhtar, Gulshan. "Indian pharmaceutical industry: an overview." *IOSR Journal of Humanities and Social Science* 13, no. 3 (2013): 51-66.

AU (African Union). Assembly of the African Union Eighth Ordinary Session 29 – 30 January (2007). Addis Ababa,

AU (African Union). "Doing business in Africa. invest in Africa 2015". (2015).: http://www.un.org/en/africa/osaa/pdf/pubs/ 2015investinafrica.pdf (Accessed 21 May 2020).

Akpan, C. P.; Archibong, I. A. and Undie, J.A. "Lecturers' access to research fund in Nigerian universities: challenges and strategies for improvement". (2010). http://socioumane.ro/blog/analesocioumane/files/2011/04/Akpan-Archibong-Undie.pdf (Accessed 10 October, 2019).

Akpochafo, W. P. "Revitalizing Research in Nigerian Universities for National Development". *Educational Research and Review* 4, No 5 (2009): 247-251.

Amuasi, J. H. "Technology Transfer and Local Manufacturing of Pharmaceuticals: The South African Case". Paper presented at the African Dialogue on Technology Transfer for Local Manufacturing Capacity of Drugs and Vaccines, held in Cape Town, South Africa, 10th – 11th December, (2009). https://www.tralac.org/images/docs/5550/amuasi-presentation-december-2009.pdf (Accessed 10 May, 2020).

AUC/UNIDO (African Union Commission & United Nations Industrial Development Organization) (2012) "Pharmaceutical Manufacturing Plan for Africa Business Plan", Addis Ababa. (2012)

Bako, S. "Universities, Research and Development in Nigeria: Time for a Paradigmatic shift". Paper prepared for the 11th General Assembly of CODESRIA, on Rethinking African Development Beyond Impasse:

Towards Alternatives, Maputo, Mozambique, 6th – 8th December, (2005).

Baro, E.E., Bosah, G.E., and Obi, I.C. "Research funding opportunities and challenges: A survey of academic staff members in Nigerian tertiary institutions". *The Bottom Line* 30, No.1 (2017): 47-64

Bello, T.O. "Funding for research in science and technology in Nigerian universities: the gender perspective". *Journal of Emerging Trends in Educational Research and Policy Studies* 3, No.1, (2015): 34-38.

Berger, M., Murugi, J., Buch, E., Ijsselmuiden, C., Moran, M., Guzman, J., Devlin, M. and Kubata, B. "Strengthening pharmaceutical innovation in Africa". Council on Health Research for Development (COHRED) and New Partnership for Africa's Development (NEPAD) (2010). http://apps.who.int/medicinedocs/documents/s18255en/s18255en.pdf (Accessed 4 October 2019).

Cele, P.C., and Lekhnaye, L.M. "Governance of the R&D productivity at the research institution based on socio-demographic indicators". *Risk Governance and Control Financial Markets & Institutions* 6, No.3 (2016): 53-59. DOI:10.22495/rcgv6i3c2art7

Chete, L. N., Adeoti, J. O., Adeyinka, F. M., and Ogundele, O. "Industrial development and growth in Nigeria: Lessons and challenges". WIDER Working Paper Series 019, (2014). World Institute for Development Economic Research (UNU-WIDER).

Delisle, H, Roberts, J.H, Munro M, Jones L, Gyorkos T.W. "The role of NGOs in global health research for development". *Health Res Policy Syst.* 21, No.3. (2005) doi: 10.1186/1478-4505-3-3. PMID: 15723694; PMCID: PMC554095.

DFID (Department for International Development) "Increasing access to essential medicines in the developing world". UK Government policy and plans. London. (2004). Department for International Development.

Dhar, B., Rao, C. N., and Gupta, V. "Transfer of Technology for Successful Integration into the Global Economy: A Case Study of the Pharmaceutical Industry in India" UNCTAD/ITE/IPC/MISC. 22, (2002) https://unctad.org/en/Docs/iteipcmisc22_en.pdf (Accessed 30 May, 2020).

Donwa, P.A. "Funding of academic research in Nigerian universities". Paper presented at the 2nd International Colloquium on Research and Higher Education Policy, UNESCO Headquarters, Paris, 29 November-1 December, 2006.

Drame, I., Connor, S., Hong, L., Bimpe, I., Augusto, J., Yoko-Uzomah, J., Weaver, S., Assefa, F., Portney, J., Gardner, S., Johnson, J., and Tofade, J. "Cultural Sensitivity and Global Pharmacy Engagement in Africa".

American Journal of Pharmaceutical Education 83 No. 4, (2019): 60—618. DOI: 10.5688/ajpe7222. PMID: 31223167; PMCID: PMC6581344.

Driskell, J.E., King, J., and Driskell, T. "Conducting Applied Experimental Research". *Laboratory Experiments in the Social Sciences* 2, (2014): 451-472. Academic press.

Economic Survey 2020-21. Government of India, Ministry of Finance, Department of Economic Affairs, Economic Division, New Delhi. https://www.indiabudget.gov.in/economicsurvey/ebook_es2021/index.html#p=471

EEC (European Economic Commission). Council Regulation (EEC) No. 1768/92 of 18 June 1992 concerning the creation of a Supplementary Protection Certificate for Medicinal Products (1992) http://eur-ex.europa.eu/LexUriServ/site/en/consleg/1992/R/01992R1768-2007 0126-en.pdf (Accessed June 8, 2010).

Egwumyenga, E.J. "Dystrophies and associated crisis in research and academic publication in Nigerian universities". *Anthropologist* 10, No. 4 (2008): 245-250.

Eisenberg, J. "Putting research to work: Reporting and enhancing the impact of health services research". *Health Serv Res* 36, (2001): x-xvii.

Ekeigwe, A. A. "Drug Manufacturing and Access to medicines: the West African story. A literature review of challenges and proposed remediation". (2019). http://doi.org/10,1186/s41120-019-0032-x

Ekpenyong, A., Udor, A., Kpokiri, E., and Bates, I. "An analysis of Pharmaceutical Workforce Capacity in Nigeria". *Journal of Pharmaceutical Policy and Practice* 11, No. 20 (2018): 1-9.

Ekwoaba, J. O., Ikeije U. U., and Ufoma, N. "The Impact of Recruitment and Selection Criteria on Organizational Performance". *Global Journal of Human Resource Management* 3, No.2 (2015): 22-33.

Federal Ministry of Health. "Medicine prices in Nigeria, Prices people pay for medicines". A publication of the Federal Ministry of Health, in collaboration with the World Health Organisation, DFID, EU and Health Action International. (2006).: https://www.afro.who.int/sites/default/files/2017-06/nigeria_medicine_prices.pdf. (Accessed 10/10/2020)

Federal Government of Nigeria (FGN) (2007). https://www.bpp.gov.ng/wp-content/uploads/2019/01/Public-Procurement-Act-2007pdf.pdf. Accessed September 27, 2022

Federal Government of Nigeria (FGN). "Executive Order No 003" (2017). https://www.nipc.gov.ng/product/executive-order-no-003-of-2017/

FMST (Federal Ministry of Science and Technology) "The National Science, Technology and Innovation (STI) Policy". Federal Ministry of Science and Technology, Abuja. (2011). http://fmst.gov.ng/uploadfil/sti_policy2011.pdf (Accessed November 9, 2021)

Federal Ministry of Health. "Draft of National Health Policy - Promoting the Health of Nigerians to Accelerate Socio-economic Development". Federal Ministry of Health (2016).

Federal Ministry of Science and Technology. "The National Science, Technology and Innovation (STI) Policy". Federal Ministry of Science and Technology, Abuja. (2011). http://fmst.gov.ng/uploadfil/sti_policy2011.pdf (Accessed November 9, 2012)

Federal Ministry of Health, Nigeria. "Access to and rational use of medicines at the household level". (2010). www.apps.who.int/medicinedocs/documents/s16887e/s16887e.pdf (accessed 17/08/2013)

FMoH- WHO (Federal Ministry of Health and World Health Organisation) "Baseline Assessment of the Pharmaceutical Sector". 2002 https://apps.who.int/iris/handle/10665/69108. Accessed 21/09/2022.

FMoH-WHO (Federal Ministry of Health and World Health Organisation) "Nigeria's National Drug Policy" (2005). https://www.health.gov.ng/doc/DrugPolicy.pdf. Accessed September 27, 2022

Geuna, A. "The Economics of Knowledge Production: Funding and the Structure of University Research". Cheltenham, UK: Edward Edgar (in Millar & Senker), (1999).

GDB (Global Burden of Disease). "Measuring performance on the Healthcare Access and Quality Index for 195 countries and territories and selected subnational locations: a systematic analysis from the Global Burden of Disease Study 2016". *Lancet* 391, (2018): 2236–2271 http://dx.doi.org/10.1016/ S0140-6736(18)30994-2

Gumel, F. "Investment Opportunities in the Pharmaceutical Sector-Nigeria/Pakistan". (2014) https://www.pwc.com/ng/en/assets/pdf/pakistan-and-nigeria-pharma-relations.pd00f. Accessed October 8, 2019.

Hofman, K., & Kramer B. "Human resources for research: building bridges through the Diaspora". *Global Health Action* 8, No.1 (2015). DOI: 10.3402/gha.v8.29559

ICRA (Indian Credit Rating Agency). "The Indian Pharmaceutical Industry". ICRA, New Delhi: (1999). <http://www.icraindia.com> (Access 25/10/2020).

Jitta, J., Whyte, S. R., and Nshakira, N. T. "The availability of drugs: what does it mean in Ugandan Primary Care"? *Health Policy Plan* 65, (2003): 167-179.

Joshi, Hemant N. "Analysis of the Indian pharmaceutical industry." *Pharmaceutical Technology* 30 (2003): 74-94.

Kaplan, W, and Laing, R. "Local Production of Pharmaceuticals: Industrial Policy and Access to Medicines: An Overview of Key Concepts, Issues and Opportunities for Future Research": https://www.who.int/medicines/technical_briefing/tbs/KaplanLocalProductionFinal5 b15d.pdf. (Accessed 25/03/20).

Kovalevaa, T. M., Khvostenkoa, O.A., Glukhovaa, A.G., Nikeryasovab,V. V., and Gavrilov D.E. "The Budgeting Mechanism in Development Companies". *International Journal of Environmental & Science Education* 11, No. 15 (2016): 7726-7744.

Lam, A. "Work Roles and careers of R&D Scientists in Network Organizations". *Industrial Relations A Journal of Economy and Society* 44, No. 2 (2005): 242-275. DOI:10.1111/j.0019-8676.2005.00383.x

Langa, P. V. "African Diaspora and Its Multiple Academic Affiliations: Curtailing Brain Drain in African Higher Education through Translocal Academic Engagement." *Journal of Higher Education in Africa / Revue de l'enseignement Supérieur En Afrique* 16, no. 1/2 (2018): 51–76. https://www.jstor.org/stable/26819628.

Malecki, E.J. and Tootle, D.M. "The role of networks in small firm competitiveness". *Int. J. Technology Management, Special Issue on Informal Information Flow*11, Nos. 1/2. (1996): 43-57.

Mansfield, E. "Basic Research and Productivity Increase in Manufacturing". *American Economic Review* 70, (1980): 863-873.

McIntyre, D., Thiede, M., Dahlgren, G., & Whitehead, M. "What are the economic consequences for households of illness and of paying for health care in low-and middle-income country contexts?" *Social science & medicine* 62, No. 4 (2006): 858-865.

McNeill, P.M., Kerridge, I.H., Arciuli, C., Henry, D. A., Macdonald, G. D., Day, R. O. and Hill, S. R. "Gifts, Drug Samples, and other Items Given to Medical Specialists by Pharmaceutical Companies". *Bioethical Inquiry* 3, (2006): 139–148. https://doi.org/10.1007/s11673-006-9019-0

Mosadeghrad, A.M. "Factors influencing healthcare service quality". *Int J Health Policy Manag*. 3, No. 2, (2014):77-89. doi: 10.15171/ijhpm.2014.65. PMID: 25114946; PMCID: PMC4122083.

Musa, S. "Ibadan University and Welfare of Nigeria, Ibadan, Nigeria". University of Ibadan 40th Anniversary Lecture. (1988).

NACETEM (National Centre for Technology Management). "Nigeria's R&D Survey 2006/07". Ile-Ife, Nigeria: NACETEM. (2011).

Nigeria and TRIPS: "Positioning Nigeria for the Promotion of a Sustainable National Development". https://www.researchgate.net/publication/313064505_Nigeria_and_TRIPS_Positioning_Nigeria_for_the_Promotion_of_a_Sustainable_National_Development (accessed Oct 09 2019).

NIRP (Nigeria Industrial Revolution Plan). Nigerian Federal Ministry of Industry, Trade and Investments. (2014) https://nationalplanning.gov.ng/wp-content/uploads/2020/12/Nigeria-Industrial-Revolution-Plan.pdfFrascasti Manual (2002), OECD. Accessed 17/10/2022.

NIRP. (Nigeria Industrial Revolution Plan). Federal Minister of Industry, Trade, and Investment, Federal Secretariat, Abuja. (2014) http://www.nipc.gov.ng/NIRP.pdf (Accessed June 9, 2020).

NOTAP (National Office for Technology Acquisition and Promotion). "National Strategy for Competitiveness in Raw Materials and Products Development in Nigeria". (2016). https://www.rmrdc.gov.ng/Techno2016Papers/NationalStrategyMain.pdf (Accessed 4 October, 2019)

NOTAP (National Office for Technology Acquisition and Promotion) "Establishment of IPTTOs" (2020) NOTAP Webpage, https://www.notap.gov.ng/content/establishment-ipttos (Accessed May 30, 2020).

Nworgu, B.G. "Educational Research: Basic Issues and Methodology". Wisdom, Ibadan. (2006).

Nyanwura, E. M., and Esena, R. K. "Essential Medicines Availability and Affordability: A Case Study of The Top Ten Registered Diseases in Builsa District of Ghana". *International Journal of Scientific & Technology Research* 2, No.8, (2013). ISSN 2277-8616 208

Obukohwo, E.O., Olele, E. H. and Buzugbe, P.N. "Assessing Efficiency in the Pharmaceutical Sector of Nigeria". *CBN Journal of Applied Statistics* 9 No. 2 (2018): 131-148. https://www.cbn.gov.ng/out/2019/std/pages%20131%20-%20148_a371_ubokohwo%20et%20al_g.pdf. Accessed 17/10/2022.

Ogaji, J.I., and Ojabo, C.E. "Pharmacy education in Nigeria: The journey so far". *Archives of Pharmacy Practice* 5, No. 2 (2014): 47-60.

Onyeji, E. "NHIS: NMA directs doctors to shun state health insurance schemes". (2018)

https://www.premiumtimesng.com/news/top-news/302357-nhis-nma-directs-doctors-to-shun-state-health-insurance- schemes.html. Accessed 12/02/2020.

Oyewale, A. A. "The Nigeria National Innovation System: Issues on the Interactions of the Key Elements". Monograph Series (No 1), National Centre for Technology Management (NACETEM), Federal Ministry of Science and Technology, Obafemi Awolowo University, Ile-Ife, (2010).

Perlitz, Uwe, Tobias Just, Martina Ebling, and Norbert Walter. "India's pharmaceutical industry on course for globalisation." *Deutsche Bank Research* (2008): 1-12.

PCN (Pharmaceutical Council of Nigeria). "Accredited Universities for Pharmacy programmes in Nigeria". (2021) https://www.pcn.gov.ng/universities-accredited-for-pharmacy-programmes-in-nigeria/

PwC (Pricewaterhouse Coopers Limited). "Sustainability of State Health Insurance Schemes in Nigeria Beyond the Launch". (2019). https://www.pwc.com/ng/en/assets/pdf/sustainability-state-health-insurance-nigeria.pdf. (Accessed 10/07/2020).

RMRDC (Raw Materials Research and Development Council). "National strategy for competitiveness in raw materials and products development in Nigeria, Competitiveness strategy". (2016). ISBN-978-978-8525-39-4.

Simpkin, V., Namubiru-Mwaura, E., Clarke, L., and Mossialos, E. "Investing in health R&D: where we are, what limits us, and how to make progress in Africa". *BMJ Global Health*, 4 (2019): e001047. doi:10.1136/ bmjgh-2018-001047.

Siyanbola, W.O., Oladipo, O.G., Oyewale, A.A., Famurewa A.J., and Ogundari, I.O. "Academia-industry interactions in Nigeria Pharmaceutical Innovation System". *Procedia - Social and Behavioral Sciences* 52, (2012) 279 – 289. Academia-Industry Interactions in Nigeria Pharmaceutical Innovation System - ScienceDirect (Accessed August 10, 2020).

Stankiewicz, R. "Academics and Entrepreneurs: Developing University-Industry Relations". Pinter Publishers, London. (1986).

Statista. "Foreign Direct Investment (FDI) Inflows in Nigeria from 2010 to 2020" (2020) Obtained from: https://www.statista.com/statistics/1302942/foreign-direct-investment-inflows-in-nigeria/ (Accessed August 17, 2022)

The Global Fund. (2019). Through https://www.theglobalfund.org/en/portfolio/country/?loc=NGA&k=430b8acd-ef36-4ef1-8231-0e730499d19a

Thomas Database. Hatch-Waxman Act Drug Price Competition and Patent Term Restoration Act of 1984, Status, Abstract and Summary from the Thomas Database: Bill (2010).

Ugbam, O.C. and Okoro, E. A. "A Strategic Study of the Nigerian Pharmaceutical Sector: Organizational Leadership, Market-share, and Competitive Performance". *International Journal of Business, Humanities and Technology* 7, No.1(2017).

UNCTAD (United Nations Conference on Trade and Development) "Investment Policy Review, Nigeria, (2009). UNCTAD/DIAE/ PCB/2008/1; https://unctad.org/en/Docs/diaepcb20081_en.pdf. (Accessed 04/10/2019).

UNECA (United Nations Economic Commission for Africa) "Review of policies and strategies for the pharmaceutical production sector in Africa: policy coherence, best practices and future prospective". Addis Ababa. © UN. (2020). https://hdl.handle.net/10855/43788

UNIDO (United Nations Industrial Development Organization)- "Pharmaceutical Sector Profile, Nigeria, Strengthening the Local Production of Essential Generic Drugs in Least Developed and Developing Countries". (2011). http://www.unido.org/sites/files/ (Accessed 30/05/2020)

UNIDO (United Nations Industrial Development Organization) "Pharmaceutical Manufacturing Plan for Africa, Business Plan". Prepared as part of the AUC-UNIDO partnership, Addis Ababa (2012). https://www.unido.org/sites/default/files/2013-02/PMPA_Business_Plan_Nov2012_ebook_0.PDF

USAID (United States Agency for International Development) (2021) Obtained from: https://www.usaid.gov/nigeria/global-hUSealth.

USAID (United States Agency for International Development) (2021). Global health. Available at https://www.usaid.gov/nigeria/global-health. (Accessed 05-08-2021).

USFDA (United States Food and Drug Administration) "Generic medicines work the same as brand-name medicines". (2021) https://www.fda.gov/drugs/generic-drugs/generic-drug-facts. Accessed 17/10/22

Varntanian, S. "The Role of RD in the modern pharmaceutical industry – Challenges and benefits". Technical report. https://www.researchgate.net/publication/331844283_The_role_of_R_D_in_the_modern_pharmaceutical_industry-challenges_and_benefits. Accessed 13/10/22.

Wakeel, A. I. and Ekundayo, P. M. "Determinants of pharmaceutical industry's performance in Nigeria". *Managing Global Transitions*14, No. 3 (2016): 267-282.

Wambebe, C., & Ochekpe, N. "Pharmaceutical sector profile: Nigeria". Vienna: United Nations Industrial Development Organization. (2011).

Wang, C., Yang, J., Cheng, Z., and Ni, C. "Postgraduate Education of Board Members and R&D Investment - Evidence from China". *Sustainability 11:* No. 22. (2019): 1-17. DOI:10.3390/su11226524

WHO (World Health Organization). "World malaria report". Geneva, Switzerland: World Health Organization, (2014).

WHO (World Health Organization). "The World Medicines Situation". (2004) WHO/EDM/PAR/2004.5.

WHO (World Health Organization) *Prequalification of Medicine*. (2005). https://extranet.who.int/prequal/content/benefits-who-prequalification

WIPO. WIPO Intellectual Property Handbook. WIPO Publication No. 489E (2004).

WIPO (World Intellectual Property Organisation). "World Intellectual Property Indicators." (2017). Geneva: World Intellectual Property Organization.

WHO (World Health Organization). "Addressing the global shortage of, and access to medicines and vaccines". Report by the Director-General. (2018). Background vol. EB142/13. Geneva: World Health Assembly, 50.

Yusuf, A.K. "An appraisal of research in Nigeria University sector". *Journal of Research in National Development* 10, No. 2 (2012): 321-330.

APPENDIX A

LIST OF ORGANISATIONS COVERED IN THE KEY INFORMANT INTERVIEWS

S/N	NAME OF ORGANISATION	Location
1.	Department of food & drug services of the federal ministry of health	Abuja
2.	WAPCP	Lagos
3.	NIROPHARM	Lagos
4.	NAIP	Lagos
5.	ACPN	Lagos
6.	PMG-MAN	Lagos
7.	AHAPN	Lagos
8.	NNMDA	Lagos
9.	NIMR	Lagos
10.	NIPRD	Abuja
11.	RMRDC	Abuja
12.	NAFDAC	Abuja
13.	PCN	Abuja
14.	PSN	Lagos
15.	NOTAP	Abuja

APPENDIX B

LIST OF PHARMACEUTICAL FIRMS COVERED IN THE STUDY

S/N	Name of Firm	State of Location
1.	AC Drug Limited	Enugu
2.	Afrab-Chem Ltd	Lagos
3.	Bioraj Pharm	Kwara
4.	Busy Bee Pharma Inds Ltd	Anambra
5.	Chris Ejik	Lagos
6.	Cinnamon Drugs Limited	Enugu
7.	Edo Pharm Ltd	Edo
8.	Emzor Pharmaceutical	Lagos
9.	Esehi Pharm Industry	Edo
10.	Evan Medical Pls	Lagos
11.	Fidson	Lagos
12.	Gauze Pharmaceutical & Labs Ltd	Anambra
13.	Greenlife Pharmaceutical	Lagos
14.	Impact Pharmaceutical Limited	Enugu
15.	Jesil Pharmaceutical	Niger
16.	Kingsize Pharmaceutical Limited	Anambra
17.	Kunmed	Lagos
18.	May and Baker Nig Ltd	Lagos
19.	Mopson	Lagos
20.	Neimeth International Pharm	Lagos
21.	Nemel Pharmaceutical Emene	Enugu
22.	Neros Pharmaceutical	Lagos
23.	New Divine Favour Pharmaceutical	Anambra
24.	Pal Pharmaceutical Nig Ltd	Kano
25.	Pax Pharmacy Limited	Anambra
26.	Service Pharm	Edo
27.	Sidom Pharmaceutical Industries Limited	Enugu
28.	Skt Pharm	Lagos

29.	Transglobe Pharmaceutical Company	Anambra
30.	Ugolab Nigeria Ltd	Kano
31.	Vitabiotics	Lagos
32.	Zolon Health Care	Lagos

Project Team Members/ List of Contributors

Engr. Prof. Okechukwu Ukwuoma	Project Co-ordinator
Prof. Wilson Erhun	Team Leader
Dr Aderonke Ayo-Lawal	Desk Officer/ Project Secretary
Dr Ayobami Oyewale	Technical Member
Dr Caleb Adelowo	Technical Member
Mr Emmanuel Ejim-Eze	Technical Member
Mrs Elizabeth Omimakinde	Technical Member
Mr Amaechi Ugwu	Project Assistant